Revised and updated

Basic
Macrobiotic
Cooking

Twentieth anniversary edition

Procedures

———

of Grain and

———

Vegetable

———

Cookery

Julia Ferré

George Ohsawa Macrobiotic Foundation
Chico, California

Edited by Carl Ferré
Illustrations by Jim North/Graphic Works
Cover design by Christy Thomas
Cover photgraphs by Debra Moon and Carl Ferré

First edition 1987
Twentieth anniversary edition 2007

ISBN 978-0-918860-59-0

Foreword

I met Julia Ferré at the Moniteau Farm Camp in central Missouri in 1980. She helped me with my cooking class, which was held in the poorly equipped farm barn. At such a class, she was a big help.

She came to our French Meadows Camp in Northern California near Lake Tahoe a year later. After the summer camp, she stayed with us at Vega Study Center as a kitchen helper. She remained and helped with my cooking classes for more than a year. Even with her busy schedule, she always found time for kindness to others, for example, baking many cookies and cakes for the Foundation staff at Christmas time.

I am very happy that her cookbook has finally materialized; this book is the first one written by one of my Vega students. This book is written by a busy, young mother who has continued to write during the time of just being married, establishing a new home, and while pregnant and nursing her first baby.

However, I am most happy with the publishing of this book because I am sure that this cookbook will be a great help to the many people who want to try this style of cooking, as well as those who have been practicing macrobiotics for some time, because it explains macrobiotic cooking thoroughly, clearly, and in easy-to-understand language.

I recommend her book highly to all macrobiotic followers, and especially for beginners.

Cornellia Aihara
November 1986

Acknowledgments

No book is a simple endeavor and the ideas in this book were molded from many individuals. I would like to acknowledge and thank my original teachers, Cornellia and Herman Aihara, plus these teachers who have influenced me directly and indirectly: George and Lima Ohsawa, Noboru Muramoto, Michio and Aveline Kushi, Jacques and Yvette DeLangre, Junsei and Kazuko Yamazaki, Annemarie Colbin, Rebecca Wood, Meredith McCarty, Christina Pirello, and Dawn Pallavi. In addition I would like to thank Kristina Turner, Wendy Esko, Lenore Baum, Barb Jurecki-Humphrey, David and Cynthia Briscoe, Rachel Albert Matesz, Margaret Lawson, Jessica Porter, Bob Carr, Lino and Jane Stanchich, Chuck Lowery, Laura Stec, Packy Conway, James Brunkow, and Suzanne Jensen for all their inspirations.

A heartfelt thanks goes to Laurel Ruggles for her precise editing work on the first edition of this book, to Bob Ruggles for his counsel, and to Sandy Rothman who originally inspired me to write this book.

Thanks to Gus, Nels, Franz, and John who continue to eat at home and give me feedback. And last, but never least, thanks and love to Carl Ferré for his help in writing the theory chapter, his input and editing for the revised edition, and for all his love and support over the years.

Preface

Many people are concerned about food. Everyone wants to be healthy and information abounds on ways to eat to have more energy. Advice ranges from "eat more veggies" to "avoid salt" and "reduce fat" to "increase fat, lower carbs." Furthermore, many people are seeking ways that food can help to prevent diseases or support in the recovery from illness.

Macrobiotics is one way to address these concerns. It is suited for anyone wanting to take care of themselves and willing to take the time and effort to learn. While macrobiotics often begins with an approach to diet that emphasizes whole grains, beans, and fresh vegetables, it includes principles that encourage flexibility and adaptability and learning how to increase self-knowledge.

Macrobiotics has been around for years, maybe as long as modern-day vegetarianism. Like vegetarianism, many misconceptions have arisen. Both are associated with severe adherence to food choices and restrictions. Other assumptions include that one must devote long hours in the kitchen or learn complicated Asian ideas. While much of the origin of macrobiotic thought came from Japan, there is no requirement one must change one's thinking or habits to Japanese customs. In fact, many people lead happy and enriched lives through the simple suggestions offered through macrobiotics without mastering Asian terms or utensils such as chopsticks.

This book seeks to open the door of macrobiotics to make it available for anyone eager to learn. Its emphasis is on cooking. Chapters are organized according to food groups. Within the chapters, information is presented by the procedures or methods of cooking. Practical information such as menu planning and how to use a pressure cooker is included, as well as theoretical information such as yin and yang and acid and alkaline.

This book grew out of my desire to see a beginning macrobiotic cookbook that anyone could use. When I began macrobiotics in 1980, I was single, worked 40 hours a week, and often lacked time or energy to cook. I would page through the available cookbooks for inspiration, but would end up preparing the same old rice and vegetables. When I studied with Cornellia Aihara, I learned different techniques and how to apply these techniques to a variety of foods.

Techniques are the procedures or methods of cooking that allow one to make a complete meal out of brown rice, pinto beans, and carrots. Techniques provide creative ideas by which one can enhance food, balance a meal, experiment. Techniques are the tools of the trade. Foods and choices of food matter, yes, but techniques make the difference. It is one thing to buy healthy food. It is another to know what to do with it. Cooking techniques provide the foundation for healthy eating.

The original *Basic Macrobiotic Cooking* was published in 1987. Four kids and almost twenty years later, I began the revision of the original text. I thought it would be simple. What I didn't foresee was that I would relearn the power of macrobiotics.

The power of macrobiotics lies in its application and whether or not it can be done easily. Dietary theories are fine, but if not practical, make no difference in anyone's life.

When I reviewed the book to see where it needed revision, I was pleasantly surprised. Typos, yes. Format changes, yes. Quantities of water or salt, additions of herbs and spices, yes. Techniques, no. The techniques needed no revisions. I am still using the cooking, cutting, and balancing techniques as written twenty years ago. These techniques have sustained and nourished me and my family with the passing years. They have provided variety for holidays, birthdays, and ever-changing tastes. What a revelation!

I am an everyday cook, preparing simple foods for my family each day. I hope you too enjoy the simple things in life.

This is an everyday cookbook. May this book offer you techniques and guidelines on your journey of taking care of yourself. And may you be blessed as you cook for yourself and your loved ones, everyday.

Julia Ferré

Contents

Grains 56

Noodles 73

Vegetables 78

Soups 104

Introduction

Once you know how to scramble eggs, you can scramble eggs, whether you have four eggs or twelve, have a different pan, or are camping. So it is with macrobiotic cooking. Once you know how to boil brown rice, make soup, or prepare vegetables, you can cook these items, whether the measures are varied, vegetables are small or large, or the utensils or stove are different.

This book is about basic grain and vegetable cookery, with an emphasis on the how-to's of cooking. There are good recipes too, of course, but to me, cooking is more than just so much of this with so much of that sautéed for so much time. Cooking is an integration of ingredients and technique. Macrobiotic cooking has a third element, a principle that helps you create order in and through your cooking. This book will give you an introduction to macrobiotic cooking—the foods, the techniques, and the principles.

The Foods – A macrobiotic approach to food is simple. It encourages a diet based on what traditional cultures or our ancestors ate. What did our ancestors eat? Whole foods. Local, seasonal foods. Foods they grew themselves. These were whole grains, beans, vegetables, fruits, nuts, and foods from the ocean such as sea vegetables and fish. Animal foods were included—more in some cultures and less in others.

A modern-day macrobiotic approach reinforces traditional diets through an emphasis on whole grains, beans, vegetables, fruits, nuts, and sea vegetables. Animal foods such as fish, poultry, red meat, and dairy are considered luxury (or in some cases remedial) foods and are included or restricted depending on individual need and preference. In this book, fish and eggs are included; red meat, poultry, and dairy are not. Most beginning macrobiotic practitioners avoid the use of red meat and dairy; however, these foods are not prohibited once one learns advanced techniques for proper selection and preparation.

In this book, some information on various foods is given in the respective chapters. For further details on specific foods, consult *The New Whole Foods Encyclopedia* by Rebecca Wood.

The techniques – A macrobiotic approach to cooking includes learning various culinary techniques. The techniques covered in this book include: boiling (cooking with water), sautéing (cooking in oil), baking (cooking with heat that surrounds food), pressure cooking (cooking with higher pressure), pickling (fermentation), marinating (penetration of flavors), cutting vegetables, and balancing meals. These are presented in simple format with sample recipes in order to teach how to apply the techniques. These techniques can be applied to a variety of foods and can be found in all cuisines and even in gourmet cookbooks.

While other techniques are found in other books, you will find information here that provides a basic foundation in grain and vegetable cookery and for further experimentation. Kitchen hints, the care and use of tools, and cutting styles found on pages 26-55 of this book are very helpful, especially to those new to cooking whole grains and fresh vegetables.

The principles – Macrobiotic principles are based on concepts that are thousands of years old. The underlying assumption is that food affects health. In practice, this means consumption of foods that sustain and nourish, and avoidance of foods that are harmful.

While complete analysis of macrobiotic principles is beyond the scope of this book, the theory chapter that follows this introduction provides a simplified explanation of yin and yang. Also included is a summary chart of acid-forming and alkaline-forming foods.

The practical application of these theories is put to use in the menu planning chapter. The recommended readings chapter provides sources for further information on macrobiotic principles and theories.

Learning macrobiotic cooking – You can delve right in and start learning about macrobiotic foods, cooking methods, and principles all at once, or you can take your time and learn at a slower pace. At the very beginning, start by cooking foods you know you will eat and use techniques you are comfortable with. Include new, unfamiliar foods and new, unfamiliar techniques as you are ready, perhaps one new food or technique per meal; if it doesn't turn out, you still have a meal. If you are using a new technique, use familiar foods at first. If you wish to prepare a new food, then use a familiar technique. In this manner you change gradually and can avoid overwhelming yourself with many new foods and techniques all at once. Thus you can assimilate the ideas and remember them better.

Making the transition – Adopting a macrobiotic approach to daily diet can be a big change, especially if many of the foods and cooking techniques are new. For simplicity, keep in mind that wholesome, whole foods are encouraged, while refined and processed foods are avoided. Try to eliminate preservatives, dyes, and artificial ingredients completely. In addition, replace:

> red meat with fowl, fish, and grains and beans in combination.
> refined sugars with fresh fruit and natural sweeteners.
> refined grains and grain products with whole grains and grain
>   products.
> canned and frozen vegetables with fresh vegetables.
> heavily sugared or salted snacks with good quality snacks of
>   wholesome ingredients.

You can make the change in two weeks or two years depending on your own preference. A gentle transition may be easier for you, your family, and friends to assimilate and accept. On the other hand your present condition may make a faster change more desirable.

How to Use This Book

How recipes are arranged – The chapters are organized by procedures rather than by recipes and thus the procedure itself is listed first. Sample recipes used with that procedure are listed second. Comments and information about that particular procedure, variations, and ideas for additional recipes are listed third.

You may wish to consult the index to find recipes for a specific item such as brown rice or winter squash. Or, you may prefer to page through the grain chapter until you reach a brown rice recipe you want to use.

Either way, make sure to read the first page of that chapter as it contains general information. Then read through the entire procedure before cooking the recipe.

Measurements – Setting out measurements is difficult. What is standard? Many factors affect how a dish will turn out. For example, I may use 2 cups of rolled oats with 5 cups of water to prepare oatmeal, yet the consistency will vary if I use a different pot, a different brand of oats, or a different stove. I may want a softer oatmeal if I'm sick or roasted oatmeal if it has been very cold and so I use slightly different measurements. Recipes were tested with the measurements as indicated both by number and by quantity. For example, one medium onion will measure 1½ cups when diced. These measurements are not meant to be hard and fast rules but rather guiding ideas from which to make adjustments.

Adapting and adjusting recipes – All the recipes can be enlarged. Most can be reduced, too. One way to adjust recipes is to use the same proportion, halving or doubling every ingredient. Another way is to change the proportions. Use two onions instead of one with the same amount of the remaining ingredients. When changing the proportions, maintain the same consistency to produce the desired end product. For example, if you have slightly more noodles than the recipe calls for and you wish to add them, add more liquid.

Recipes can be adapted by substituting ingredients. The focus of this book is on procedures and not on ingredients. Substitute similar foods in any procedure to make new recipes. Try almond butter in place of tahini, collards rather than kale, or red beans in place of pinto beans. You can create many exciting dishes by following the basic procedures and substituting ingredients.

Note on fats and oils – It is important to use quality oils and to use them in ways that are healthy. New information about fats has been discovered since the first publication of this book 20 years ago. Then, I used corn oil in baking. I don't recommend it anymore. Corn oil requires high heat and technological processes—refinements that degrade oil's fragile nature. In addition, oil processed from corn often comes from genetically modified (GMO) corn. Canola oil and safflower oil are inferior oils for these same reasons and should be avoided.

Oil is fragile. All vegetable oils except coconut oil and palm oil denature in temperatures in excess of 240 degrees. Heat, often exceedingly high, is used in the extraction and refining of most oils on the market. Chemicals are used by many manufacturers that increase the oil's shelf life and flavor, but that results in a less-than-healthy product. Labels don't always detail the full processes; it is important to be informed. Unrefined organic oils are preferred to ensure that no GMOs or chemicals are used. Oils that I currently recommend for cooking are the same ones that have been used throughout history—light and toasted organic, unrefined sesame oil; organic extra virgin olive oil; and organic, unrefined coconut oil. Other organic and unrefined oils such as flax, avocado, or walnut are valuable used unheated in salad dressings or drizzled on food.

In addition to choosing quality oils, it is important to subject oil to low temperatures only. If sautéing or frying, one must avoid heating the oil to too high of a temperature, or to the point where oil begins to smoke. Personally, I prefer olive oil and light sesame oil for sautéing vegetables and for use in grain dishes. I bake and fry with coconut oil as it can withstand higher temperatures.

Some macrobiotic practitioners avoid all baked and fried foods and thus avoid any oil subjected to high heat. My children are unwilling to take this step. If I don't provide quality baked and fried foods, they eat junk food away from home. Baked and fried foods are delicious and a part of modern cuisines everywhere. Be informed about fats and oils and choose quality organic oils for daily use, using them in ways that are healthful for yourself and those you cook for. For more detailed information about specific oils, consult Rebecca Wood's *The New Whole Foods Encyclopedia*.

Estimating numbers of servings – It is difficult to spell out exact quantities in terms of numbers of servings because serving sizes and appetites vary. The recipes in the book have no set numbers of servings; only approximate yields in terms of cups or number of muffins. The yield will vary depending on your measuring, the size of the vegetables used, and the temperature of the stove. Variations from ½ cup to 1 cup of water, a small bunch to a medium bunch, or medium-low heat to low heat can affect the yield. So yields and numbers of servings are always approximate.

Intuitive cooking – Many people cook without measuring at all, choosing to prepare meals with whatever is on hand and using a pinch of this or a pinch of that. This is an exciting way to cook and helps one to become a sensitive and intuitive cook. Once you learn techniques of cooking and employ simple menu planning and balance ideas, this type of cooking becomes a joy. This cookbook may be used as a springboard to develop the intuitive ability.

No matter how much you study and practice cooking, there is always more to discover. I hope this book will help you in your cooking and will inspire you to keep on learning.

Theory

Underlying principles – There are other diets that include whole grains and fresh vegetables. A macrobiotic diet is different in that it incorporates more than just food. There are principles underlying one's diet that help one understand how food, among other things, affects our bodies and minds. Two of these principles are the order of the universe and the unifying principle as defined by George Ohsawa, a modern-day promoter of macrobiotics.

One aspect of the order of the universe is that everything happens in an orderly way. Planets, land forms, histories of peoples, sickness, health, emotions: all things follow a definable and understandable order. The assertion is that if we align with this order, our health and well-being will be better. The unifying principle of yin and yang provides one means to help accomplish this goal.

Yin and Yang Theory

Yin and yang as tools – Yin and yang are the tools that can help us to see orderliness and thus help us to create order in our lives. Yin represents expansiveness; yang represents contractiveness. These characteristics interact with each other to define phenomena.

Yin and yang as descriptive words – Yin and yang are descriptive words to help classify and categorize. They are meaningful only when used to describe or compare things. Just as light and heavy are relative words, so yin and yang are also relative words. For example, wood is heavy compared with paper but light compared with rock. In the same way, vegetables are yang compared with fruit but yin compared with animal foods. Thus any item can be either more yin or yang depending on what it is compared with, or depending on the category.

Yin and yang and change – It is important to note that things them-selves continually change, and the conditions acting upon things also change. What is yin at one time may be yang at another, depending on many factors such as season, age, size, and location of growth.

Macrobiotic thinking is based on the idea that each person and each person's condition is unique due to a unique set of factors, and that these factors are continually changing. Thus it is preferable to learn processes and procedures rather than memorizing sets of rules and lists of recipes.

Yin and yang and harmony – We experience yin and yang factors in our lives and then determine how to use other yang and yin factors to harmonize our present condition. For example, after eating something salty, one becomes thirsty. If you study how to determine your own condition, you can then use yin and yang to help create and maintain harmony in your life. This can be done through many activities, one of which is eating.

Yin and yang and their importance to diet and cooking – We eat each day. As yin and yang factors change from day to day, our choice of food and preparations can harmonize these changing factors. When the situation changes again, the food and preparation also need to change. Cooking is a practical and daily way to apply yin and yang.

By following the simple guideline of "consume mostly grains and vegetables," you remain near the middle of the yin-yang spectrum. By eating mostly foods in the middle of the spectrum, it is easier to balance yin and yang.

Applying the theory of yin and yang to cooking – It is natural to follow the principle of yin and yang without a necessarily conscious decision. For example, when it is cold, you desire warming things. And when it is hot, you want cooling things. Simply observing yin and yang at work is a good way to begin understanding these principles.

To intentionally apply the principle of yin and yang, here are four general ideas to keep in mind.

- We need both yin and yang; the harmony of yin and yang is desired.
- It is easier to balance moderate yin and yang than extreme yin and yang.
- We become what we take in: If I eat mostly yin food, I become more yin.
- We can balance a condition by what we eat: I take in yin to help balance a more yang condition.

Classifying yin and yang – The classification of yin and yang can be applied to all of life The following examples represent some of the yin and yang qualities of foods.

Composition:

more yin	more yang
rich in potassium	rich in sodium
more watery	less watery (more dry)

Growth:

more yin	more yang
vertical growth above ground	vertical growth below ground
horizontal growth below ground	horizontal growth above ground

Size:

more yin	more yang
bigger	smaller
larger leaves	smaller leaves

Season and climate:

more yin	more yang
grown in summer	grown in winter
grown in warmer climate	grown in colder climate

Manner of production:

more yin	more yang
grown with chemical fertilizers	organically grown

Note that a carrot grown in a warmer climate is more yin than a carrot grown in a colder climate. However, such a "yin" carrot is still more yang than a tomato even if the tomato is grown in a colder climate because tomatoes as a category are more yin than carrots, as shown in the next section.

Yin and Yang of Foods and Preparations

Food categories – Foods can be categorized from yin to yang based on the ratio of yin and yang elements. The following spectrum gives a comparison of how food groups relate to each other in terms of yin and yang. This is only a general guide, as many factors influence yin and yang characteristics. Each category may overlap one or more of its neighbors. For example, some vegetables are more yin than some beans.

more yin   more yang

| oils | fruits | beans | vegetables | grains | animal foods | salt |

Each food group can likewise be categorized from yin to yang.

Grains:
more yin   more yang

| corn | oats | barley | brown rice | wheat | rye | millet | buckwheat |

Vegetables:
more yin   more yang

| tomato | cucumber | cabbage | squash | onion | turnip | carrot |

Beans:
more yin   more yang

| split peas | pinto beans | lentils | chickpeas | azuki beans |

Food groups can be further categorized from more yin to more yang. This is a good way to learn the yin and yang of foods. Here's an example to get you started.

Root Vegetables:

more yin					more yang
red radish	turnip	daikon	rutabaga	carrot	burdock

Preparation categories – We can classify the methods of preparation as more yin or more yang. Again yin and yang are comparative words. Sautéed is yang compared with boiled but yin compared with baked.

more yin					more yang
raw	boiled	pressure cooked	sautéed	baked	pickled

Raw – Food that has not been altered by cooking or pickling.

Boiled – The water boils and steam goes up and out (expansion). Also included in this category are simmered, steamed, parboiled, and blanched.

Pressure cooked – Foods are subjected to higher pressure than normal atmospheric pressure. Foods become more condensed (yang).

Sautéed – The hot oil seals in nutrition and flavor (this factor is more yang); but oil itself is considered more yin. Also included in this category are stir-fried, pan-fried, and deep-fried.

Baked – Foods are surrounded by dry heat that condenses them. Also included in this category are roasted (top of stove or oven) and broiled.

Pickled – Foods are not cooked, but are changed through pressure, salt, and length of time. Thus the yin and yang qualities are also changed depending on the amount of pressure and salt, and the length of time. Included in this category are natural pickling methods utilizing salt. Pickles made with vinegar are considered more yin, as vinegar is classified as a yin ingredient.

Additional factors – Preparations in each general category change in their yin and yang relationships to each other as other conditions such as time, amount of salt, and amount of water change.

Time: more time is more yang.

more yin	more yang
30 minute pickles	3 day pickles
vegetables baked 30 minutes	baked 1½ hours

Salt: more salt is more yang.

more yin	more yang
vegetables sautéed with a pinch of salt	sautéed with ½ tsp salt
salad with no salt	salad with a dressing including soy sauce

Water: more water is more yin.

more yin	more yang
2 cups rice and 8 cups water	2 cups rice and 3½ cups water
pickles made in salt brine	pickles made by pressing with salt

Yin and Yang of Cooking

When cooking and planning meals, there are four basic ways of combining the various yin and yang factors of foods and preparations to create harmonized dishes and meals.

Food balancing food – Use yin foods and yang foods to balance each other. Avoid having many yin items or yang items without an appropriate balance, such as a meal with only yin items. Some examples of food balancing food are grains (more yang) and vegetables (more yin); fish (more yang) served with lemon (more yin); and sea vegetables (more yin) cooked with soy sauce (more yang).

Preparation balancing preparation – Use yin preparations and yang preparations to balance each other. Avoid meals with all items prepared in only one manner, such as a meal with all baked dishes. Use at least two preparations, such as pressure-cooked food with sautéed food, or baked food with raw food.

Preparation balancing food – Use yin preparations for yang foods; yang preparations for yin foods. This method of balancing is particularly useful when preparing foods with strong yin or yang qualities, such as fruit, fish, or vegetables in the nightshade family. Some examples are baked fruit (yin food with yang preparation), steamed fish (yang food with yin preparation), tomato sauce cooked by a waterless method for a long time (yin food with yang preparation), or baked potatoes (yin food with yang preparation).

Four-way balance – Most cooking falls into this category since this method incorporates the other three methods of balancing. It involves preparing a whole meal with balanced items. Some examples are pressure-cooked rice (both more yang) with simmered vegetables (both more yin), baked fish (both more yang) with raw salad (both more yin), or boiled buckwheat (yin-yang) with sautéed cabbage (yang-yin).

Other balance considerations – While it is important to know how to balance yin and yang of foods and preparations, there may be other factors to balance. Sometimes there is a specific health condition that requires the balance of foods and preparations be more yin or more yang. In addition, it is important to recognize that foods affect acidity and alkalinity in the body. Here is a useful chart:

yin acid-forming foods	yin alkaline-forming food
grain sweeteners	beverages
oil	fruit
nuts	sea vegetables
beans	seeds
some grains	most vegetables
most grains	some root vegetables
fish	some sea vegetables
	salty soy products
	(miso, soy sauce)
	sea salt
yang acid-forming foods	yang alkaline-forming food

The study of yin and yang can be a lifelong project. But you don't have to learn yin and yang in depth in order to cook good food. What is intended here is an introduction. Menu planning is a practical place to start, see pages 259-266.

Kitchen Hints

Timetable

Time flow – Plan what to serve, and work in an orderly way.

> Allow enough time to cook. Give yourself a comfortable margin; either count backward from serving time, or count forward from when you can be in the kitchen. See general timing, which follows.
>
> Put water on to heat when preparing dishes that require boiling water.
>
> Determine which dish needs the longest time and start preparing this dish first. Approximate the cooking time for various dishes, and include the preparation time for vegetables, the soaking time for sea vegetables, the standing time for grain or pressure cooker returning to normal pressure, the cooling time for quick breads, and the setting time for kanten.
>
> Cook quicker dishes last so whole meal is done at the same time.
>
> Start tea when meal is served, so it simmers and steeps during the meal and will be hot when you are ready to serve it.
>
> Measure and soak any grains and/or beans for the next meal.

General timing – In order to have everything prepared by a certain time, estimate the time required to prepare a meal based on four general categories. Note: Increase timings if beans are boiled.

> At least 2 hours – Preparing a meal that includes pressure-cooked beans, any hard-kerneled grains, and/or baked vegetables.
>
> At least 1 hour – Preparing a meal that includes thin-kerneled grains; grains that are cut, rolled, or creamed; most soups, and/or most sea vegetable dishes.
>
> At least 30 minutes – Preparing noodles, incorporating or mixing leftovers into a new dish such as rice salad.
>
> At least 10 minutes – Reheating leftovers.

Allow more time for preparation of the following foods or prepare at times other than meal prep.

> Breads – Let rise 2 to 24 hours.
> Pickles – Ferment 2 to 4 days.
> Soaking beans and grains – Soak for 4 to 8 hours.
> Sesame seed condiments – Roast seeds and grind condiments. Allow 1 hour.
> Desserts such as pies, crisps, or cobblers – Bake for 1 hour or more and cool 2 or more hours before serving.

Cooking Hints

Top of stove or in the oven – Cooking on the top of the stove uses less energy than cooking in the oven because a smaller area is heated. When preparing a small amount of food, use the top of the stove. Roast seeds and nuts, heat leftovers, and toast bread in a skillet. Heat store-bought or homemade mochi in a covered skillet over low heat. Use the oven when baking breads, vegetables, or desserts, or when preparing many foods at the same time to make the maximum use of the space and the heat generated.

Boiling water – Put water on to heat as the first thing when entering the kitchen to cook. It will then be hot when needed, and will save time when bringing a dish to boil. When adding boiling water to a hot pan, add slowly and gently to avoid scalds. Pour away from yourself. When adding water to a pan that has layered food, pour water slowly over a spoon to avoid disturbing the layers.

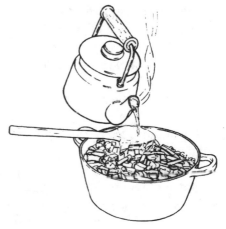

Heat – Use the appropriate heat for the pan and the specific dish. Higher heat cooks food quicker than lower heat, but is hard on the pans and can burn the food. Use:

> High heat for short cooking times. Use at the beginning of cooking to heat up pan or to bring food to cooking temperature.
> Medium-high to medium heat to bring food to a good cooking temperature. Medium-high is preferable to high because it is more gentle on pans.
> Medium-low to low heat once the pan is hot and the food is cooking well. Low heat can be used to keep food simmering for the remainder of the cooking time.
> Very low heat for long cooking times of over 1½ hours. Usually used with a heat diffuser.

Use of cover – Covers are used on pans for most cooking. Use a cover to hold the heat and steam inside, and thus cook the food faster. Use a cover to control spatters when pan-frying in oil. After cooking, use a cover on top of the pan to condense the steam and help lift food off the bottom of the pan. When all the food has been removed, soak pan with 1 inch of water and a cover on top to help make the pan easier to clean, especially if scorched.

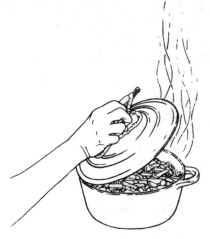

Leave the cover ajar to help prevent spillover when cooking oatmeal, beans, or other foamy foods. Remove the cover near the end of cooking for some sautéed dishes or sauces to help evaporate extra water. Lift the back edge of pot covers first so the steam goes away from you, and thus avoid steam burns.

Preparing to Sauté – Heat the pan over medium heat before adding oil. Stainless steel pans heat in 5 seconds; cast iron and enameled ware heat in 15 seconds. Add oil to the heated pan and tilt pan to spread oil, then add vegetables. Vegetables will cook quickly and not just absorb oil.

Sautéing Vegetables – Vegetables are added to pan one kind at a time, usually beginning with onions and garlic, if used. Sauté onions until color changes, that is, the opaque white color becomes transparent. The time required for this change varies with the size of the pan and the number of onions. One onion may become transparent in 1 to 2 minutes while 5 onions may take 5 to 7 minutes. Add other vegetables and sauté until the color changes or the vegetables begin to condense.

Serving proportions – Serving proportions vary with preference and choice. Proportions can change. A proportion of 2 parts grain to 1 part bean may appeal one day while a 3-part grain to 1-part bean may appeal another. If you have specific recommendations from a counselor, follow those guidelines, otherwise develop your own intuition about proportions.

Approximate sizes of servings for a meal including rice, vegetables, seeds, soup, pickles, and tea are shown in the following list.

    Rice – 1 to 1½ cups
    Vegetables – ¾ to 1 cup
    Roasted seeds – 2 Tbsp
    Soup – 1½ cups
    Pickles – 1 Tbsp
    Tea – 4 oz

Examples of servings of other items are:

    Dry condiment – 2 tsp
    Bean dish – ½ to ¾ cup
    Noodles – 1½ cups
    Sea vegetable dish – ¼ cup
    Bread – 2 slices
    Fish – 2 to 4 oz
    Dessert – ⅛ of a 9-inch pie or ½ cup applesauce

When serving each plate, enhance colors by arranging foods to make it look attractive. Use garnishes to add flavor and color. Tan grain with a tan sauce looks more appealing when scallions are sprinkled on top. Fried fish looks inviting when accompanied by a half-round slice of lemon or a sprig of parsley.

Buying Food

Buy foods you will use. Buy the best quality grains and beans you can find, such as whole, unpolished, organically grown, and free from preservatives. Buy seasonal vegetables whenever possible, locally grown if available. Flours should be freshly ground and tofu and tempeh freshly made, or as fresh as possible.

Buy undyed, untoasted sea vegetables. Fertile eggs from free-ranging birds are preferred. Buy organic, unrefined oils as suggested on pages 16-17.

Buy unrefined, mineral sea salt. Use unpasteurized and aged soy sauce and miso; pasteurization kills beneficial bacteria. Buy undyed umeboshi with no preservatives added. Bancha twig tea should be roasted and made from older twigs and leaves.

First-time shopping list – If you are starting from scratch, use this list as a guideline. The grains on this list will feed 2 people for 6 to 8 days.

> 2 pounds short grain brown rice
> 1 pound rolled oats
> 1 pound millet
> 1 pound whole wheat macaroni or other pasta
> 1 pound lentils or split peas
> ½ pound almonds or sunflower seeds
> 1 bottle organic and unrefined light sesame oil
> 1 bottle unpasteurized soy sauce
> 1 package two-year-old unpasteurized barley miso
> 4 ounces unrefined sea salt
> 1 package bancha twig tea
> 1 package kombu sea vegetable
> 1 jar tahini
> vegetables and fruits such as onions, carrots, cabbage, celery,
>   broccoli, greens, winter or summer squash, garlic, apples, and
>   pears as desired

Storing Food

Grains, flours, beans, seeds (uncooked) – Keep in airtight covered containers in a cool place at room temperature. They can be refrigerated for long storage or if in a hot climate. Place bay leaves in the containers to discourage bugs. Use flours within a week of purchase or grinding; they lose flavor and nutritional value as they sit. Use seeds within 2 months as they can become rancid. Grains and beans will keep 6 to 8 months.

Vegetables and fruits – Keep vegetables in a cool place. Onions and winter squash will keep in a cellar if whole and free from any cuts or bruises. Store squash so they don't touch each other, and turn them occasionally. Most vegetables and fruits keep well in a refrigerator. If bunches have twist-ties or bands, remove them before storing. If the vegetables are wet, allow them to dry before storing so to prevent rot. Spread on a paper bag and leave at room temperature until dry.

Generally, roots keep longer than greens. Keep in vegetable crisper or plastic bag in the refrigerator and use while still crisp. If vegetables are refrigerated as is, they tend to dry out. Some vegetables such as lettuce, scallions, and mushrooms keep well in cotton bags. Others, such as celery, keep better in plastic or in an airtight container. Parsley keeps well standing in a jar of water in the refrigerator.

Tofu and tempeh – Tofu is available in bulk or in packages. Tofu will keep refrigerated up to 7 days covered completely with water. Change water every other day. If the tofu smells bad, it has spoiled. Tempeh is often packaged; sometimes it is only available frozen. Keep in the refrigerator until ready to use, within 7 days, or in the freezer for up to 2 months.

Fish and eggs – Buy fish as fresh as possible. If your only option is frozen fish, thaw in refrigerator. Use all fish within a day of purchase. Fresh fish can be stored on ice if desired. For longer storage, sprinkle lemon juice over fish and freeze. Eggs will keep in the refrigerator for 1 month. Keep in the carton.

Oils and nut butters – Keep in a cool, dark place to prevent rancidity. Refrigerate in hot weather or if not used within 1 month.

Sea salt, miso, soy sauce, and umeboshi – Keep sea salt in a dry place. It will keep for years. Natural sea salt has no additives and may cake. Keep miso in a cool place or refrigerator. If miso has been kept a long time and a white mold forms on top, it shows that the miso is unpasteurized. This mold can be mixed in or scraped off.

Keep soy sauce in glass in a cool place. If you buy a large quantity, such as a gallon, and keep it for over a year, white flecks may float to the top. The flecks do not harm the soy sauce but show that the soy sauce is unpasteurized. The soy sauce can be strained and used. Keep umeboshi plums and paste in a cool, dry place. They will keep a long time; if kept over a year, they will dry somewhat and the salt may crystallize. They can still be used.

Sea vegetables, arrowroot, kuzu, bancha tea, herbs and spices – Keep in a dry place, avoiding a sunny window or a warm spot such as above the stove. Keep herbs and spices in covered containers and use within one year of purchase. Bancha twig tea, arrowroot, and kuzu will keep for over a year while sea vegetables will keep two or more years. To prevent these items from absorbing moisture, they can be stored in glass or waterproof containers.

Cooked foods – Cooked foods, except fish and eggs, will keep at a cool room temperature until the next meal. Remove from cooking pans, place in bowls, and cover with a bamboo mat or basket so air can circulate but food doesn't dry out. If the container is tightly covered, the food may spoil. Grains and tea will keep one to two days unrefrigerated.

Cool foods to room temperature before transfering to containers and placing in the refrigerator. Keep in covered containers to prevent drying out or absorbing smells. Soup and tea keep well in glass jars.

Tools: Care and Use

Outfitting Your Kitchen

In addition to common kitchen tools such as pots and pans, bakeware, mixing bowls, and spoons, the following tools are of great help.

Vegetable brush – Different types of natural bristle brushes are available. Some have a handle; some are held in the hand. Use only with clean water; avoid soap. Vegetable brushes can be used to clean bamboo mats and suribachi.

Knives – A rectangular Japanese knife is ideal for cutting vegetables as it is lightweight and gives a clean, crisp cut. Use a serrated knife for cutting bread. A small paring knife is handy for coring foods but slow when chopping on a board.

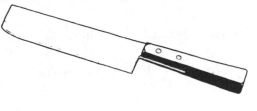

Pots and pans – Use stainless steel, cast iron, Pyrex, ceramic, or enameled cookware. Aluminum cookware is not recommended as aluminum can react with food and leave traces of aluminum in the food.

Pressure cooker – This can be a big investment, but it is well worth it because a pressure cooker can provide a lifetime of service. There are various kinds and sizes. Buy stainless steel or enameled ware rather than aluminum. Inquire about replacement parts when buying. Parts for some brands are hard to find.

Heat Diffuser – Sometimes re-
ferred to as a flame tamer, this
is a flat metal disc with punched
holes. It is placed between a
pan and the burner to spread
the heat and help keep the food
from sticking to the bottom of
the pan and burning. It works
well with a pressure cooker.

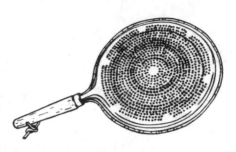

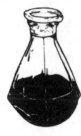

Soy sauce dispenser – There are different types
of glass containers designed to dispense soy sauce
drop by drop. Some soy sauce is sold in small dis-
pensers. A glass screw-on cap will last longer than
a plastic one.

Tea strainer – Strainers made of bamboo or ceramic are used to strain
tea when serving. Clean with a vegetable brush and avoid soap.

Japanese grater – This kind of grater shreds the food very finely so
that juice can be extracted from the shreds. Available in Oriental food
stores or through mail order, it may be of porcelain or metal.

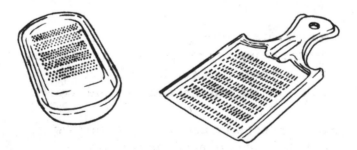

Miscellaneous items – These specialty items are useful: Suribachi and
suricogi, Japanese mortar and pestle used to blend food; Japanese pickle press; Foley food mill; and hand or electric flour mill.

Pots and Pans

Heavy pans – Heavy pans have thick walls and bottoms. Often they are made of cast iron, enameled cast iron, or enameled steel. Heavy pans take a longer time to heat than light pans, yet they hold the heat better and can be used for longer cooking times. Waterless cooked vegetables and dishes that require a long cooking time such as soups, grains, and beans cook well in heavy pans and will not be as likely to burn.

Light pans – Light pans have thin walls and bottoms. Often they are stainless steel. Aluminum pans are light, but aluminum leaches into the food, so don't use them. Stainless steel pans heat quickly and are good when cooking dishes which require a short cooking time such as simmered vegetables, noodles, and quick soups. They tend to scorch if used for long cooking times, so place a heat diffuser underneath.

Extreme temperature changes – Avoid exposing any pan or utensil to extreme changes of temperature. Avoid putting hot pans in dishwater; cool first. Avoid adding cold water to a hot pan. Use boiling water, or cool the pan first and then add cool water.

Burned pans – Slight scorches are easy to take care of. After the dish has finished cooking, remove the pot from the burner, but do not remove the food from the pot. Let the pot stand with the cover on for 10 to 15 minutes. The steam will condense and lift the food at the bottom so all the food can be mixed together. Grains respond especially well to this method and a slight scorch can even add flavor.

If pan is burned, remove all food and discard inedible part. Soak the pan in cold water overnight with the cover on. If the burn is stubborn, boil uncovered with 2 tablespoons baking soda in 1 inch of water for 15 minutes; then soak covered overnight. Gently scrub off. To avoid burns, use lower heat, time carefully while simmering, cook in a pan appropriate for the dish, and use a heat diffuser for longer cooking times.

To bring sparkle back to stainless steel pans, clean inside and outside with 1 tablespoon lemon juice, fresh or bottled.

Cast Iron Ware

Seasoning – Non-enameled cast iron utensils must be seasoned to coat the metal so the pan can be used without rusting or imparting a metallic flavor. The initial seasoning takes 1 to 2 hours and can be repeated whenever desired. Cast iron pans improve with age.

Remove the wax finish from American-made pans before seasoning. First, wash pan in hot soapy water, rinse well, and towel dry. If using a gas stove, place over a medium flame. If using an electric stove, place the pan in a 350-degree oven to heat. Heat until all the finish has smoked off; it will take 10 to 15 minutes. Turn on a fan and open the doors. Cool 5 minutes. Coat inside and outside with a very thin coating of cooking oil such as coconut oil. Place over flame or in the oven again, and heat to settle the oil into the pan. This will take 5 to 7 minutes; the pan may smoke. Cool. Coat the inside again. Heat another 5 to 7 minutes to settle the oil into the pan. The pan is then ready to use.

If the pan gives a metallic flavor after the initial seasoning, sauté an onion in it and discard the onion. Wash the pan in hot soapy water, rinse well, heat, and oil. It is better to season a Dutch oven in an oven than on top of the stove. Heat and oil both the pan and the lid; however, don't put the lid on the pan while heating or they will seal together.

Washing and using – If the pan has been used for dry roasting you don't need to wash it. For other types of cooking, wash in clean water without soap, gently removing all visible food with an abrasive pad. Then place 1 inch of water in the pan and bring to a boil. This boiling will release any food that may be sticking to the pan. Discard water and any remaining food residue. Rinse in hot water and wipe dry. Return to burner to dry completely and coat lightly with oil to reseal. This way of cleaning will help your cast iron ware last and is especially important during the first months of use.

Cast iron pans are ideal for sautéing vegetables, toasting nuts and seeds, dry roasting grain and flour, and pan-frying fish and burgers. If used for soups or watery dishes, the food may pick up a metallic flavor, especially if the pan is new.

Miscellaneous Kitchen Utensils

Enameled cookware – Be careful not to chip the enamel with metal implements or abrasive pads. Don't dry-roast grain, flour, nuts, or seeds in them since the dry heat may crack the enamel. Avoid extreme temperature changes; especially avoid adding cold water to a hot pan as this may crack the enamel.

Knives – Use a kitchen knife only for its intended purpose; don't use it to pry up lids or cut paper, wood, or string. When cutting vegetables on a board, take care to cut only the vegetable, not the board, to help keep the knife sharp. When removing vegetables from the board, use the back of the knife to pick up vegetables or to push them off the board. Don't scrape the sharp edge of the blade across the board as this will dull the blade. After using a knife, wash and dry it immediately and put it away in a knife rack or holder. A sharp knife works better and is safer to use than a dull one; sharpen as often as necessary by any desired method. After sharpening, wash the knife to remove any oil or particles of metal. For use cutting vegetables, see pages 45-46.

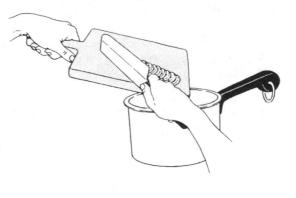

Cutting board – Hold the knife properly, and cut straight down to get a clean cut without needless cutting of the board. After using, clean the board by scrubbing both sides with a vegetable brush and clean water. Avoid soap as the board may absorb it. After cutting fish, rub lemon into the board to remove odors; then scrub with brush and clean water. Dry the board completely so it will not absorb water and become warped or cracked.

Wooden and bamboo utensils – Avoid soaking wooden utensils as they may swell and warp. Wash and rinse well. Wash bamboo baskets, mats, and strainers if food gets stuck to them. Use vegetable brush and clean water. Avoid soap.

Using a Pressure Cooker

There are many types of pressure cookers available on the market, both domestic and imported. Models range in size and material. Choose stainless steel or enameled stainless steel rather than aluminum and buy a size that fits your needs.

Cooking with pressure – A pressure cooker has an airtight seal, making possible a pressure inside the cooker greater than the atmospheric pressure outside the cooker. Foods cook quickly and condense from this strong pressure. Learning to use a pressure cooker well involves becoming familiar with your cooker and learning how to recognize full pressure.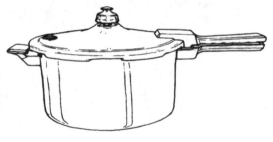

Vent/value – All cookers have a vent or value in the lid to monitor pressure. It is important that it is clear so the correct pressure will be maintained. If the vent clogs, pressure can build up, and the pressure relief plug may pop out. Check hole before placing lid on cooker to make sure vent is clear. Insert a wire or a pipe cleaner to clean if needed.

Weight – On some pressure cookers, there is a removable weight that fits on top of the vent. It controls and maintains pressure. When the sealed cooker is being heated, the weight keeps all the steam inside and the pressure increases. When up to full pressure, the steam and pressure are strong enough to jiggle the weight. When the weight jiggles, some steam escapes along with some pressure. Gentle rocking shows that there is full pressure, and also that any excess pressure is being released.

Gasket – The gasket is a rubber ring which fits in the cover of all types of cookers and creates a tight seal so the cooker can reach full pressure. Before putting the ring in the cover, make sure that both ring and cover are clean of any particles. The ring may shrink or become hard in time and should then be replaced. If the cooker doesn't reach full pressure, or if there is leakage from between the cover and the pot, you may need a new ring.

Plug – The pressure relief plug is made of rubber and it, or some other means of releasing pressure, is a safety device found on all pressure cookers. It may be under or opposite the handle of the cooker. If the pressure becomes too high (usually due to a clogged vent), the plug is designed to pop out and release the pressure before it becomes dangerously high. The plug may harden in time. If there is leakage from the plug hole, the plug may need to be replaced. The plug and the gasket are often replaced at the same time.

Bringing to full pressure – Place ingredients in the cooker. Check the ring and fit it into the lid. Check the vent to make sure it is clear. Lock the cover on the cooker. Place the weight on the vent. Place the cooker over medium to medium-high heat. Pressure will increase.

Check your owner's manual for how your specific pressure cooker will show full pressure. Some cookers have a gauge that rises with increased pressure. Others rely on sound. With this type, when the pressure becomes stronger, the cooker will begin to make noise which will increase with increased pressure. At full pressure the noise peaks, and the weight gently rocks. It will take 10 to 30 minutes to reach full pressure, depending on the quantity of food. Rocking of the weight and noise signal full pressure, not dangerous pressure. Rocking of the weight signals that steam is escaping from the vent, which is a good sign. For safety reasons, always stay in the kitchen when a pressure cooker is going up to pressure.

Cooking at full pressure – When the cooker reaches full pressure, re-move from heat. Place a heat diffuser on the burner and set the cooker on it. If cooking vegetables or soup, omit the heat diffuser and just turn down the heat. Turn the heat to low or medium-low, enough to maintain pressure. Start timing. Keep full pressure for the full cooking time, not allowing pressure to go up or down.

The secret of good pressure cooking is to get the cooker to full pres-sure and keep it there for the full cooking time. Train your ear and eye to recognize your cooker's sign of full pressure so that you know the correct time to reduce heat. For cookers with a gauge, keep the gauge at the full pressure level. For cookers that rely on sound, observe the noise level. The noise should be steady, although quieter than the peak noise and accompanied by steam escaping the vent and gentle rocking of the weight. If the weight isn't rocking, gently tap; if there is some hissing and steaming, everything is fine. If there is no steam or noise and if the heat has been very low, the pressure has probably dropped. If 15 or more minutes of cooking time remain, turn up the heat to increase the pressure. If the heat has been high, see precautions below.

Precautions – While the cooker is at full pressure, it is important to stay nearby in case a high-pressure situation occurs. Take precaution if the gauge reaches too-high a level or the cooker makes a peaking noise for a second time, signaling too-high a pressure. Remove the cooker from the burner for 3 to 4 minutes or until the gauge lowers or the weight rocks normally. Then return the cooker to the burner and set the heat lower.

Take precaution if the heat has been high and if, when tapping the weight, there is no noise or steam. This can signal that the vent is clogged or that there is not enough liquid in the cooker. Remove cooker from heat and run water over the lid to reduce pressure completely. Remove the weight and lid. Check the vent and clean it if it is clogged. Add liquid to the cooker if necessary. Return lid and weight. Continue cooking.

Leakage – If steam or foam escape from between the cover and pot, the seal is not tight. This may be caused by the cooker not being properly closed, food stuck to the gasket or to the top of the pot, or the gasket getting old and not fitting snugly. Reduce the pressure completely by running cold water over the lid. Remove the cover. Check the gasket and top of the pot for any stuck food, and clean if needed. Refit the gasket in the cover. Replace the cover, close completely, and resume cooking. If foam still comes out, the gasket does not fit snugly and should be replaced.

If foam comes out from the vent, the cooker may be too full. A little foam is not unusual, but if there is so much that it covers the lid, the vent may clog and create a problem. Watch carefully. If steam comes out with the foam, the vent is open. Beans often produce foam.

Removing the cover – Let the pressure drop completely before removing the weight and cover. This is important. Let stand until the pressure drops, or run cold water over the lid, especially when cooking vegetables. When there is no steam or noise when tapping the weight, remove the weight, and then the cover.

Cleaning and storing the cooker – Remove the gasket from the lid and wash separately. Clean the weight and the vent hole if clogged. When storing, keep the cover unlocked to avoid damaging the gasket.

Safety rules
– Cook appropriate foods only. Avoid foods that may clog the cooker (soybeans, split peas, rolled oats, and fruit).
– Soak those foods that may clog the cooker if unsoaked (whole oats, barley, beans).
– Fill cooker no more than two-thirds full.
– Check vent hole to make sure it is open before cooking. While cooking, keep in mind that the vent must be clear or the cooker may reach too-high a pressure. Steam escaping from the vent signals that the vent is open and is normal.
– Pay attention while cooker is going up to pressure. Stay nearby.
– Turn down heat at the right time.
– Remove cover only when pressure is down and the weight is off.
– Never immerse a pressure cooker at full pressure in cold water. Reduce pressure by allowing pressure to drop or by running cold water over the lid.

Using a Suribachi

A suribachi is a ceramic bowl with unglazed grooves. A suricogi is a wooden pestle. Together, they are used to blend food. The groves assist in crushing food, especially when grinding sesame seeds. Suribachi come in various sizes. Use a size large enough so the ingredients do not spill as you grind.

Placement of the bowl – Place the bowl in one of three places: On
the floor in a corner of
the room, kneel and sit on
your heels and wedge the
bowl firmly into the corner
with your knees; on your
lap as you sit in a chair; or
on a table at a good working height, the suribachi
placed on a towel to avoid
slipping.

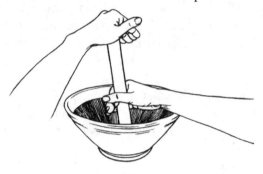

Holding the suricogi – Hold suricogi (pestle) with both hands, one near the bottom and one near the top. The bottom hand guides the suricogi all around the bowl, crushing and blending ingredients. The top hand holds the top of the suricogi as still as possible. It can also add and control weight.

Grinding – Vary the strength of grinding depending on the food being ground, the placement of the bowl, and any weight added by the top hand. Grind lightly when crushing seeds or mixing ingredients. Grind strongly when grinding salt or when making a fine mixture. It is easy to grind strongly when the bowl is on the floor and wedged into a corner.

Cleaning – An easy way to clean the grooves is to pour hot water or broth around bowl to loosen clinging ingredients. Remove and add to soup. Then wash bowl in clean water with a vegetable brush; avoid soap.

Cutting Vegetables

Cutting vegetables is a creative outlet in cooking. A cook can use different cutting styles in an individual dish or over the whole meal for variety and for appeal. In addition, cutting vegetables is a practical way to produce meals. Cutting allows different vegetables to be combined in the same dish so they can cook in the same time. Also, cutting can be used to save time, as small cuts cook faster than large cuts.

Using vegetables – Generally, younger vegetables are more tender than older ones. Also, smaller vegetables are more tender than larger ones. Use tender vegetables in salads, or in dishes which cook in a short time. Use older and larger vegetables in dishes which require longer cooking times such as soups, beans, or vegetable dishes. Some vegetables such as celery and greens come in bunches with both small and large pieces. Separate small and large pieces for various uses—small tender pieces of celery in salads, large pieces in soups.

Sizes and shapes of cuts – Use larger cuts for stews which simmer an hour or longer and for vegetables which will be served alone as a side dish, like winter squash. Young tender vegetables, which cook quickly, should be cut in large pieces to prevent them from overcooking.

Use smaller cuts for most soups, grain dishes, and vegetable combination dishes. Larger, older vegetables will cook more thoroughly if cut in small pieces.

Use a different cut for each vegetable in a dish. Don't use all rounds or all dice cuts, but allow the cuts to complement one another. Matchsticks and crescents go well together as do mince and quarter-rounds. Rounds and matchstick look awkward together, but large crescents and "logs" look appealing. Vary cuts for different vegetables used in the same meal. Use both large cuts and small cuts; similar large pieces for a side dish and similar small pieces for soup.

When cutting, notice that some vegetables require different cuts for different parts: The stems of greens are often cut into thin rounds, while the leaves are often cut into squares; broccoli flowers and stems are cut differently. Some vegetables vary in their dimensions: A carrot is wider at the top than the bottom. When cutting quarter rounds, cut the top into thinner cross cuts and the bottom into thicker cross cuts so all pieces will cook evenly. Celery varies in that the inside stalks are more tender and can be cut into larger pieces while the outside stalks are more tough and are best cut into thinner or smaller pieces. Bunched vegetables such as scallions vary in size: Cut smaller scallions into larger sizes and larger scallions into smaller sizes when used in the same dish.

Cutting protocol – Flavors of different vegetables can mingle on the cutting board, and strongly flavored vegetables like onion and garlic can change the flavor of another vegetable. Cut one kind of vegetable at a time. Remove from board into a bowl until ready to cook, or cut vegetables in the order of use and put them directly into the pot. Wipe the board and knife with a clean sponge (no soap) between different kinds of vegetables, especially for vegetables used in different dishes.

Using a Knife

Rocking Method – Upon purchasing a rectangular vegetable knife, I began to cut vegetables following various cutting diagrams shown in cookbooks. I held the vegetables with fingers out. I held the knife loosely at the end of the handle and cut by rocking the knife, keeping the front of the knife on the board and using the back of the knife to cut. The cut used a down, back stroke. It took a long time to cut vegetables, and the pieces were uneven.

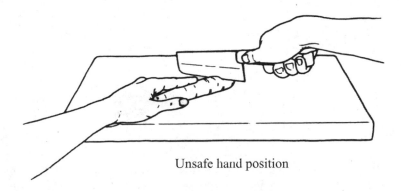

Unsafe hand position

Whole knife method – In cooking classes, Cornellia Aihara used a different method of cutting. She cut fast and evenly. She held the vegetables with curled fingers, using the tips of the fingers and nails

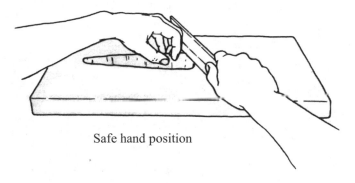

Safe hand position

to keep the vegetables from moving and to protect the fingers. In this way, the upper part of the knife blade comes in contact with the knuckles, and the cutting edge is far from the fingertips. After each cut, the knuckles move back ever so slightly, measuring the distance of the next cut.

Cornellia held the knife differently, too. She held it firmly and grasped the knife at the junction where metal meets handle. This way of holding the knife allows more control when cutting. To cut, the whole knife is picked up, and then sliced down on a forward stroke. The upper arm and body move forward with this cut, and the blade meets the board evenly.

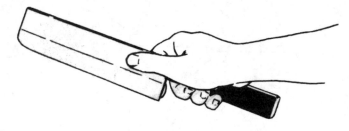

Learning this whole-knife cutting was awkward for me and gave me cramps for a few days. After ten days, it was comfortable; and in one month, I was cutting faster and more consistently. If you desire, learn this method by practicing slowly.

Cutting Styles

Minced onions

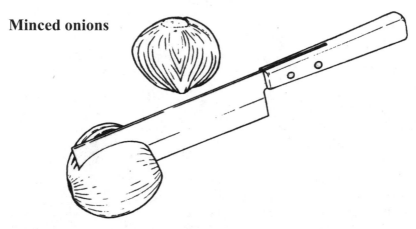

1. Slice onion in half lengthwise.
2. Place one half on board, cut side down, root end farthest from knife.
3. Slice cuts into the onion, leaving onion together at root. Leave just enough to keep onion together. This connection makes the next step easier.

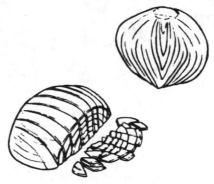

4. Slice across the cuts.
5. When you get to the uncut part, cut as necessary in order to mince.
Note: Cuts can be close together for fine mince or farther apart for large mince.

Crescents

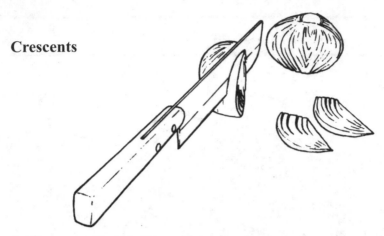

1. Slice vegetable in half lengthwise.
2. Hold one half with cut side away and root up.
3. Slice vertically with a piece of the root in each slice.
4. Rotate vegetable on its axis for the next slice. Each slice will be like a small wedge. Slices may be thick or thin.

Note: Any round vegetable can be cut in crescents.

Flowers

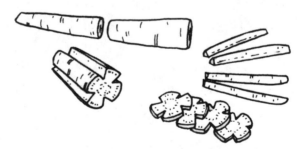

1. Cut vegetable into 3- or 4-inch sections.
2. Make 3 or 4 V-shaped cuts along the length of the vegetable.
3. Slice across.

Note: Pieces can be thin or thick.

Rounds

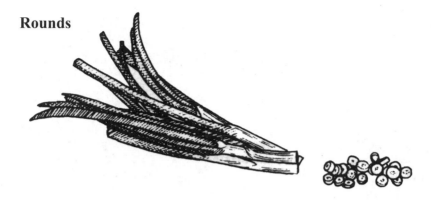

Slice across vegetable, thin or thick as desired.

Half and quarter rounds

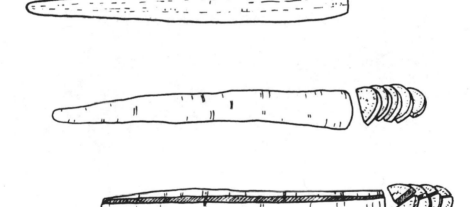

1. Slice vegetable in half lengthwise. For quarter rounds, slice each piece lengthwise in half again.
2. Place cut side down.
3. Slice across.
Note: Pieces can be thin or thick.

Diagonals

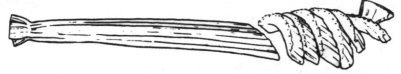

Slice diagonally across the vegetable, adjusting the length of the diagonal
by the angle of the cut, and making thin or thick pieces as desired. Hold
the knife perpendicular to the board.

Chunks

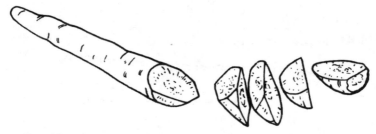

1. Place vegetable with stem end closest to knife.
2. Cut a thick diagonal cut.
3. Roll vegetable 90 degrees towards you.
4. Cut another thick diagonal.
5. Roll again and cut. Pieces will have 3 to 4 cut edges.
Note: Make long diagonals farther apart for larger chunks.

Matchsticks

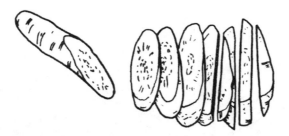

1. Slice vegetable into diagonals.
2. Overlap diagonal slices, if they haven't fallen into position when cut.
3. Slice diagonals lengthwise into matchsticks.
Note: Pieces can be thick or thin, as desired. Pieces can also be long or short, depending on the length of the diagonals. Each diagonal can be cut individually, but it takes longer than when pieces overlap.

Shaved

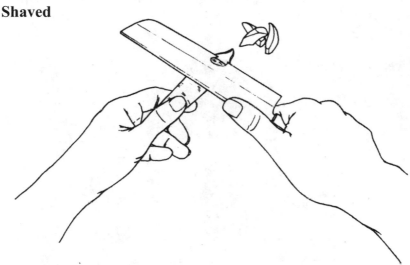

1. Hold vegetable in your hand straight away from your body.
2. Shave the vegetable by cutting away from the body as if sharpening a pencil or whittling.
Note: Shavings can be long or thick as desired. This cutting style is often used for burdock root, carrot, or other long root vegetables.

"Logs" or "paper cut"

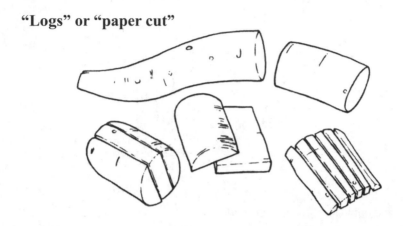

1. Slice vegetable across into 2- to 3-inch long sections.
2. Slice each section into vertical slabs.
3. Slice each slab into vertical rectangles.
Note: Very thin rectangles look more like sheets of paper while thick rectangles look more like logs.

Diced or minced

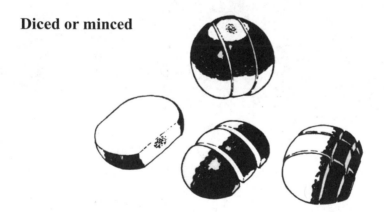

1. Slice vegetable lengthwise into vertical slabs.
2. Slice each slab into vertical logs.
3. Slice across the logs, thin or thick as desired.
Note: This dice cut can be varied to make cubes or thin squares. Minced pieces are very small. This cut can be used on round or long root vegetables.

Cubes

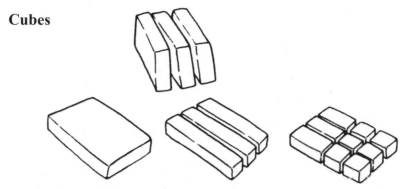

1. Cut tofu into slabs.
2. Cut each slab into logs.
3. Cut each log, or set of logs, into cubes.
Note: Cubes can be large or small.

Squares, squash

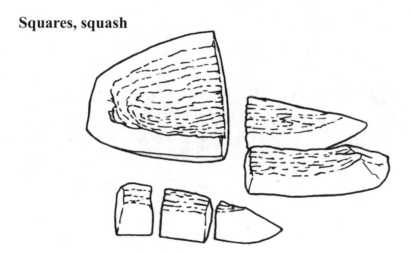

1. Cut stem from squash.
2. Slice squash lengthwise.
3. Remove seeds with a metal spoon.
4. Slice one half into lengthwise pieces.
5. Slice lengthwise pieces into squares.
Note: One side of each square will have skin. Squares can be large or
    small.

Squares, greens

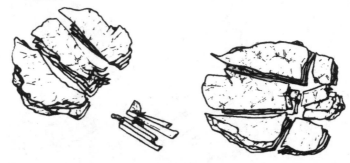

1. Place greens flat on top of each other. Notice where the leaf and stem meet. All these junctions should be on top of each other. This causes the bottoms of the stems to be uneven with each other, but will make the greens easier to cut.
2. Cut the stems as desired—rounds are often used, or discard.
3. Slice leaves into lengthwise pieces.
4. Slice across the pieces into squares.
Note: Squares can be large or small. This works well with "flat" greens such as collard greens or mustard.

Shredded

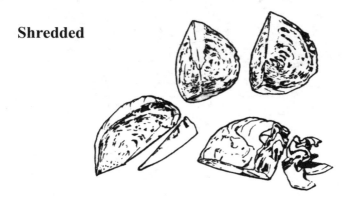

1. Cut cabbage into 4 wedges; crescent cut.
2. Remove core.
3. Place on board with cut side down.
4. Slice thinly across leaves.
Note: Shred is a fine cut. Cut fine or very fine. To shred leafy greens, follow steps 1 and 2 for squares, above, then cut thinly across the leaves.

Cored

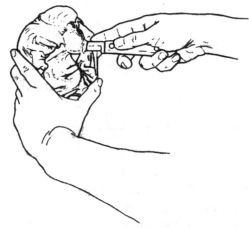

1. Hold the whole vegetable on a flat surface, core up.
2. Cut all around core with a strong paring knife, angling knife toward the center of the cabbage.
3. Remove core by lifting out. It will be pointed.

Flowerets

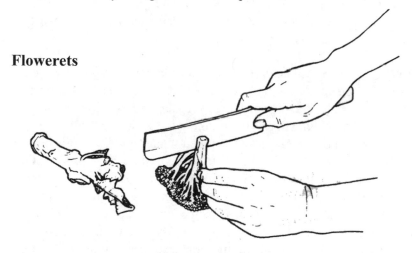

1. Cut broccoli below the flower at whatever length is desired.
2. Hold the flower on the board with the stem pointing up.
3. Cut into the stem toward the flower, but cut only the stem.
4. Divide the flower by pulling gently with your fingers.
Note: For cauliflower, remove the hard bottom stem. Place stem side up and divide by cutting into the stem, as above.

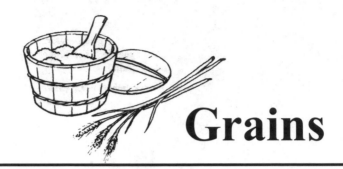

Grains

Use – Whole grains, used by people all over the globe and cultures throughout history, are a fundamental food in macrobiotic cooking. Whole grains contain both bran and germ and provide more nourishment than refined grains. From hard-kerneled grains such as whole oats and rye to thinner-kerneled grains such as millet, grains have been the basis for humans' food supply for eons.

Washing – Wash grains prior to cooking because some dust settles on the grain during the milling process. Measure grain into cooking pan. Add water, swirl, and drain. Repeat 2 times or until the rinse water is clear.

Soaking – Soaking whole grains is a vital step that allows them to cook thoroughly. Dried grains have enzyme inhibitors—natural preservatives that allow the grains to be stored for many years. These inhibitors, however, interfere with digestion. Soaking the grains neutralizes the effect of these inhibitors. Grain swells when soaked and the inside of each kernel softens, which is the first step in preparing grain for sprouting. Soaking activates the germ of the grain and increases nutrient availability. And, grains that are soaked before cooking taste more delicious.

Soak whole grains such as brown rice, oats, wheat, rye, and barley for 4 to 8 hours for best results. Adjust the soaking time for the season with shorter soaking time in summer and a longer soaking time in the winter. Millet, quinoa, and buckwheat, along with cut or creamed cereal grains cook more quickly than the hard-kerneled grains. Although I usually don't soak any of these grains or grain products, some sources recommend it. If there is no time for soaking, roast grains first. Roasting inactivates the enzyme inhibitors and enhances flavor.

Sea Salt – Sea salt is alkaline-forming for the body and helps balance acid-forming grains. Sea salt adds flavor—grain tastes sweeter than without sea salt. For grains that are soaked, add sea salt after soaking, just before cooking.

Cooking times – Generally, cook hard-kerneled grains longer than soft-kerneled grains or grains that are cut, rolled, or creamed. Within the times specified, the longer cooking times produce a more soft and creamy grain.

> *Brown rice, whole wheat, whole rye, whole oats, whole and pearled barley* – 45 minutes to 2 hours. These hard-kerneled grains need to be soaked before cooking.

> *Buckwheat, millet, wild rice, cracked wheat, steel-cut oats, flaked (rolled) grains, polenta, quinoa, amaranth, teff, and creamed cereals* – 30 minutes to 1 hour.

> *Couscous, bulgur, and pastas* – 5 to 15 minutes.

Heat – Use medium to medium-high heat to bring grains to full pressure or to a boil. Then reduce heat as directed. For longer cooking times, use a heat diffuser under the pot to prevent burning.

Cooking – Let grain cook; avoid lifting the cover or stirring while cooking. If the cover is removed and the grain is stirred, steam escapes which causes heat loss, and the grain will not cook completely. After cooking, remove pan from burner and let stand for 5 to 10 minutes with cover on. The steam will lift the bottom grain from the pan so it can be mixed with the rest of the grain.

Mixing – After grain is cooked and allowed to stand 5 to 10 minutes, mix with a dampened wooden spoon or rice paddle. Slip spoon between grain and the side of the pan, going all around the pan. Gently but thoroughly mix grains from top to bottom.

Cleaning the utensils – Soak cookware, utensils, and bowls in cold water 5 to 10 minutes to remove any sticking kernels. Then wash in hot water.

Boiled Grain, Soaked

Procedure – Wash and drain grain. Soak for the desired time in the full quantity of water. Add sea salt after soaking. Cover. Bring to a boil. Simmer over low heat for the time indicated, using a heat diffuser if needed.

Brown rice, short or long grain – Soak 4 to 8 hours. Simmer 1 hour. Yield: 6 cups for short rice; 6½ cups for long.

2 cups brown rice
4 cups water
⅛ tsp sea salt

Barley – Soak 4 to 8 hours. Simmer 1½ hours. Yield: 4 cups.

1 cup barley
4 cups water
pinch sea salt

Porridge, whole oats or rice – Simmer for 1½ to 2 hours. Yield: 4 or more cups.

1 cup whole oats or short grain brown rice
4 cups water, or more
pinch sea salt

Comments – This procedure is recommended for hard-kerneled grains. For variety, mix grains (such as rye and rice, or barley and oats) and cook with 2 cups water to 1 cup grain. If unable to soak, roast grain first as on page 62.

Boiled Grain, Unsoaked, Hot Water

Procedure – Bring water to a boil. Add sea salt, then grain. Cover. Return to a boil. Simmer over low heat for the time indicated, using a heat diffuser if needed.

Kasha (roasted buckwheat groats) – Simmer 25 minutes. Yield: 7 cups.

> 4 cups water
> ⅛ tsp sea salt
> 2 cups kasha

Bulgur – After adding bulgur, cover and return to a boil, then remove from heat and let stand 40 minutes or until liquid is absorbed. Fluff and serve. Yield: 6 cups.

> 3 cups water
> ⅛ tsp sea salt
> 2 cups bulgur

Couscous – After adding couscous, cover and return to a boil, then remove from heat and let stand 5 to 10 minutes or until liquid is absorbed. Fluff and serve. Yield: 6 cups.

> 2½ cups water
> ⅛ tsp sea salt
> 2 cups couscous, whole wheat or refined

Millet – Wash and drain before cooking. Simmer 25 to 30 minutes. Yield: 8 cups.

> 2 cups millet
> 6 cups water
> ⅛ tsp sea salt

Comments – This procedure and the next are recommended for grains that have thin kernel walls and for cut, rolled, and creamed grains. Both procedures are used with the same grains, cooking times, and number of utensils. However, the grains cook differently. In this hot water method, the grain is added to boiling water and tends to swell only slightly because it is immediately surrounded by hot water. For example, rolled oats become more fluffy. In the cold water method, everything is mixed together first, and the grain tends to swell more as it comes to a boil. Rolled oats become creamy.

Boiled Grain, Unsoaked, Cold Water

Procedure – Place grain, cold water, and sea salt in a pan. Bring to a boil. Cover. Simmer over low heat for the time indicated, using a heat diffuser if needed, with lid ajar for grains that tend to boil over.

Oatmeal – Simmer 20 minutes. Yield: 5 cups.

> 2 cups rolled oats
> 5 cups water
> ⅛ tsp sea salt

Steel-cut oats – Simmer 35 minutes. Yield: 6½ cups.

> 2 cups steel-cut oats
> 6 cups water
> ⅛ tsp sea salt

Wild rice – Simmer 50 to 60 minutes. Drain excess water when done. Yield: 4 cups.

> 1 cup wild rice
> 4 cups water
> ⅛ tsp sea salt

Millet with quinoa or amaranth – Wash and drain before cooking. Simmer 25 to 30 minutes. Yield 8 cups.

1¾ cups millet
¼ cup quinoa or amaranth
6 cups water
⅛ tsp sea salt

Polenta or rice cream – Bring 2 cups polenta or rice cream and 4 cups water to a boil, stirring constantly until thickened. Add 2 cups more water and "push" water between cereal and bottom of pan to help prevent scorching. Simmer polenta 30 minutes, or rice cream 45 minutes, over a heat diffuser. Yield: 7 cups for polenta; 6 cups for rice cream.

---

2 cups polenta or coarsely ground brown rice
6 cups water
⅛ tsp sea salt

Comments – This procedure is recommended for whole grains that have a thin kernel wall and for grains that are rolled or cut. Coarsely ground grains such as brown rice or wheat make delicious creamed cereals. If you have a home flour mill, grind your grain fresh. Roast for more flavor, page 62.

For variety, mix grains and flakes. Try oatmeal with buckwheat or rye flakes; or millet with steel-cut oats. Another variation is to add other ingredients to simmer with the grain, such as minced onion, winter squash, or cauliflower with millet; raisins with oatmeal; or chopped scallions to polenta during the last minutes of cooking.

In addition, leftover cooked brown rice can be added and boiled with the simmering grain. Add ¼ to ½ cup cooked brown rice to 2 cups polenta.

Boiled Grain, Roasted

Procedure – Bring water to a boil. Place grain in a separate pan (see comments) and dry roast (no oil) over medium heat for 2 to 10 minutes, stirring constantly, until fragrant and lightly browned; whole grains will pop. Mix roasted grain, boiling water, and sea salt in a pan. Bring to a boil. Cover. Simmer over low heat for the time indicated, using a heat diffuser if needed.

> **Brown rice** – Wash and drain before roasting. Simmer 1 hour, using a heat diffuser. Yield: 6 cups for short rice; 6½ cups for long rice.

2 cups short or long grain brown rice
4 cups water
⅛ tsp sea salt

> **Buckwheat** – Simmer 30 minutes. Yield: 7 cups.

2 cups buckwheat
4 cups water
⅛ tsp sea salt

> **Teff** – Simmer 15 minutes. Yield: 3 cups.

1 cup teff
3 cups water
pinch sea salt

> **Amaranth** – Simmer 10 minutes. Yield: 1½ cups.

1 cup amaranth
1 cup water
pinch sea salt

Quinoa – Wash well before roasting. Simmer 15 to 20 minutes. Yield: 4 cups.

1 cup quinoa
2 cups water
pinch sea salt

Polenta or rice cream – After roasting, remove pan from heat. Add 4 cups boiling water, and whisk to smooth lumps. Add 2 cups additional water around the edge of pan, using a spoon to "push" water between cereal and the wall and bottom of pan. This water will help prevent scorching. Return pan to heat and cover. Bring to a boil and simmer 30 minutes for polenta or 45 minutes for rice cream, using a heat diffuser. Stir well and serve. Polenta can be set into a loaf pan for frying later, page 252. Yield: 6½ cups for polenta, 6 cups for rice cream.

2 cups polenta or coarsely ground brown rice
6 cups water
⅛ tsp sea salt

Comments – This procedure can be done in two ways. One way is to add boiling water to roasted grain; the other is to add roasted grain to boiling water. I like to roast in cast iron ware or stainless steel, and to prepare various grains differently. For example, I roast polenta in a Dutch oven and add boiling water to it, but I roast buckwheat in a skillet and add it to boiling water.

Roasting the grain before boiling adds flavor. Teff, buckwheat, bulgur, polenta, millet, and rice cream are especially enhanced when roasted, but any grain or coarsely ground cereal can be roasted. For variation, add minced onion and simmer with the grain. Or, add minced scallions during the last 2 minutes of cooking.

Boiled Grain, Sautéed

Procedure – Bring water to a boil. Heat oil in a separate pan and add grain. Sauté until fragrant, stirring constantly. Add boiling water and sea salt. Cover and bring to a boil. Simmer 30 minutes over low heat, using a heat diffuser if needed.

Buckwheat or bulgur – Yield: 7 cups for buckwheat; 6 cups for bulgur.

4 cups water
1 tsp light sesame oil or olive oil
2 cups buckwheat or bulgur
¼ tsp sea salt

Polenta or millet – See page 63 for polenta preparation. Wash and drain millet before sautéing. Yield: 6½ cups for polenta; 8 cups for millet.

6 cups water
1 tsp light sesame oil or olive oil
2 cups polenta or millet
¼ tsp sea salt

Comments – Sautéing grain in oil before boiling adds even more flavor. Any grain may be sautéed, but these examples are especially recommended. These examples are simple but can be varied with the addition of herbs. Add granulated garlic or curry powder to bulgur, flaked basil or cinnamon to millet, or experiment with your favorite seasonings.

Boiled Grain with Sautéed Vegetables

Procedure – Bring water to a boil. Heat oil in a separate pan and add vegetables, one kind at a time, in the order listed. Sauté each kind briefly. Add grain. Sauté until fragrant, stirring constantly. Add boiling water and sea salt. Cover and bring to a boil. Simmer 10 to 30 minutes over low heat, using a heat diffuser if needed. See page 63 for polenta preparation.

Polenta, millet, or quinoa with onion – Simmer 30 minutes. Yield: 6¾ cups for polenta; 8½ cups for millet or quinoa.

6 cups water for polenta or millet; 4 cups water for
    quinoa
1 tsp light sesame oil or olive oil
1 medium onion, minced, 1½ cups
2 cups polenta, millet, or quinoa
¼ tsp sea salt

Polenta with green pepper – Simmer 30 minutes. Yield: 7½ cups.

6 cups water
1 tsp light sesame oil or olive oil
1 medium onion, minced, 1½ cups
1 medium green bell pepper, diced, ¾ cup
2 cups polenta
¼ tsp sea salt

Bulgur with mushrooms – Simmer 10 minutes or until water is absorbed. Yield: 7 cups.

4 cups water
1 tsp light sesame oil or olive oil
1 medium onion, minced, 1½ cups
12 medium mushrooms, diced, 2 cups, ¼ pound

2 cups bulgur
¼ tsp sea salt

Comments – This procedure allows creativity and can be great fun. What vegetables would you like to enhance your grain dishes? How about quinoa with onion, celery, and carrot; or couscous with onion, broccoli, and carrots. Herbs and spices lend themselves well to this procedure. Add and sauté with the vegetables to spread the flavor throughout the dish; for example, onion, garlic, curry powder, green beans, carrot, and couscous. While the examples here use faster cooking, thinner-kerneled grains, this method also can be used for brown rice and other grains that require longer cooking times.

Boiled Grain, Layered with Vegetables

Procedure – Bring water to a boil. Heat oil in a separate pan and add vegetables, one kind at a time, in the order listed. Sauté each kind briefly. Add ¼ cup boiling water. Layer grain over vegetables. Cover. Steam 5 minutes. Add remaining boiling water without disturbing layers. Add sea salt. Cover and bring to a boil. Simmer 30 minutes over low heat. Mix to serve.

Millet with vegetables – Yield: 9½ cups.

6 cups water
1 tsp light sesame oil or olive oil
1 medium onion, minced, 1½ cups
1 medium stalk celery, diced, ¾ cup
1 small carrot, thin quarter rounds, ½ cup
2 cups millet, washed and drained
¼ tsp sea salt

Kasha with vegetables – Yield 8 cups.

---

4 cups water
1 tsp light sesame oil or olive oil
½ medium onion, minced, ¾ cup
1 medium stalk celery, diced, ¾ cup
1 medium carrot, thin quarter rounds, ¾ cup
2 cups kasha
⅛ tsp sea salt

Comments – Layering grain over sautéed vegetables produces a light and fluffy dish. The grain won't stick to the pan because the vegetables are on the bottom. Try other grain and vegetable combinations such as millet or polenta layered over onions and winter squash. Grains may be roasted before layering for additional flavor and variety.

This procedure is similar to Layered Vegetables with Cornmeal, page 85. Vary the proportion of grain to vegetable for desired end, whether primarily a grain dish or mainly a vegetable dish.

Grain to Water Ratio for Boiled Grain Dishes		
Grain	**Water**	**Yield**
1 cup amaranth	1 cups	1½ cups
1 cup barley	4 cups	4 cups
1 cup brown rice	2 cups	3 cups
1 cup buckwheat	2 cups	3½ cups
1 cup bulgur	2 cups	3 cups
1 cup couscous	1¼ to 1½ cups	3 cups
1 cup millet	3 cups	4 cups
1 cup oatmeal	2½ cups	2½ cups
1 cup polenta	3 cups	3¼ cups
1 cup quinoa	2 cups	4 cups
1 cup teff	3 cups	3½ cups
1 cup wild rice	4 cups	4 cups

Pressure-Cooked Grain

Procedure – Wash and drain grain. Soak for the desired time in the full quantity of water. Add sea salt after soaking. Lock cover on pot. Set pressure according to pressure cooker instructions. Place cooker over medium-high heat. Bring to full pressure. Slip a heat diffuser under the cooker and turn heat to low. Cook at full pressure for the time indicated. See pages 38-41 for further information on using a pressure cooker.

Short or long grain brown rice – Soak 4 to 8 hours. Pressure cook 40 to 45 minutes. Yield: about 10 cups.

> 4 cups brown rice
> 5 to 6 cups water
> ¼ tsp sea salt

Barley, whole oats, whole rye, or whole wheat – Soak 4 to 8 hours. Pressure cook 45 minutes. Yield: 5½ cups for rye; 6 cups for others.

> 2 cups barley, whole oats, whole rye, or whole wheat
> 4 cups water
> ¼ tsp sea salt

Brown rice combinations – For the second ingredient, use barley, millet, long grain brown rice, sweet rice, wild rice, whole oats, whole rye, or whole wheat. Soak 4 to 8 hours. Pressure cook 45 minutes. Yield: 6½ cups for rye; 7 cups for others.

> 2 cups short grain brown rice
> ½ cup other grain
> 4 cups water
> ¼ tsp sea salt

Brown rice and bean combinations – Use azuki beans, black soybeans, chickpeas, kidney beans, or mung beans. Soak 8 hours with rice and kombu. Salt is not used in this recipe. Pressure cook 45 minutes. Yield: 13 to 13½ cups.

---

4 cups brown rice
½ cup beans
7 cups water
4-inch piece of kombu

Millet – Millet does not need to be soaked, but does require more water than the standard proportion. Pressure cook 20 minutes. Can be set into a loaf pan for frying later, page 252. Yield: 7 cups.

---

2 cups millet
5 cups water
⅛ tsp sea salt

Rice Porridge – Soak 4 to 8 hours. Pressure cook 1 hour. Yield: 7 cups.

---

2 cups brown rice
6 cups water, or more as desired
⅛ tsp sea salt

Porridge – Use any desired grain or grain combination listed above. Pressure cook with 3 or more times the amount of water and a pinch of sea salt for the times listed above for the specific grain.

Comments – Pressure cooking is a thorough way to cook whole grains that have a hard kernel. It is generally not called for when cooking buckwheat, or grains that are cut, flaked, or creamed. Most hard-kerneled grains pressure cook better when soaked first. If there is no time for soaking, roast grain first. Place washed and drained grain in a skillet and dry roast over medium heat until browned, fragrant, and beginning to pop. Then place in pressure cooker with water and salt and proceed as above.

The amount of water, grain, and sea salt varies with the size and condition of the pressure cooker and the quantity of grain being cooked. Use the proper sized pressure cooker for the amount of grain. In a 4-to-6-quart pressure cooker, cook at least 4 cups grain; smaller amounts do not cook well. Use a 2-quart (1.8-liter) size for 2 to 3 cups grain.

If you wish to cook 1 or 1½ cups grain and only have a large pressure cooker, use a covered bowl or Ohsawa Pot, a specialized ceramic pot available from *www.goldminenaturalfood.com*, inside the pressure cooker: Place 1 cup rice soaked in 1½ cups water in a Pyrex dish or measuring cup, stainless steel bowl, or Ohsawa pot with ⅛ teaspoon sea salt. Place cover on bowl. Fit the bowl into the cooker. Place 2 cups water in the bottom of the pressure cooker. Pressure cook as directed in the standard procedure. This yields 3 cups of cooked rice. For 4 cups of cooked rice, use 1½ cups uncooked rice and 2 cups water.

When cooking brown rice, use a proportion of 1 cup rice to 1¼ cups water for firm rice. Use 1 cup rice and 1½ cups water for a softer, but still firm rice. For other hard-kerneled grains (wheat, rye, barley, and whole oats), use 2 cups water per 1 cup of grain. Use ¼ teaspoon of sea salt for 4 cups of grain. Kombu can be used in place of salt and is recommended when cooking grain and bean combinations. Use 1 inch of kombu per 1 cup of grain.

When cooking, a certain amount of water changes to steam and evaporates. A new pressure cooker has a very tight seal and less water evaporates than with an older pressure cooker. It is possible to use a proportion of 1 cup water per 1 cup rice in a new cooker for firm rice. Remember to cook an appropriate amount for the size of the pressure cooker as stated above.

Baked Grain

Procedure – Bring water to a boil. Wash and drain grain. Roast grain in a separate dry skillet (no oil) until fragrant, stirring constantly, 5 to 10 minutes. Place roasted grain, sea salt, and boiling water in a casserole dish. Cover. Bake for the time indicated at 350 degrees.

Brown rice – Bake 1 hour. Yield: 10 cups.

> 6 cups water
> 3 cups brown rice
> ⅛ tsp sea salt

Millet – Bake 30 minutes. Yield: 8½ cups.

> 6 cups water
> 2 cups millet
> ⅛ tsp sea salt

Comments – Baking roasted grain produces a pilaf-type dish suitable for colder weather and holiday menus. Use boiling water and covered ovenware for proper and thorough cooking. For variation, sauté vegetables and bake with the grain. For example, sauté onion, carrot, shiitake mushroom, and burdock and bake with roasted brown rice. Serve with roasted sunflower seeds.

Rice Balls

Procedure – Cut one sheet of nori into 12 squares. Dampen hands. Press cooked rice into a ball. Make a hole in the center. Place pitted umeboshi plum in the hole. Press again to close hole. Cover ball with 2 pieces of nori, partially covering the rice ball.

Rice ball

> 2 pieces cut nori
> ½ cup cooked brown rice
> ½ small umeboshi plum, pitted

Comments – Rice balls are a traditional Japanese food prepared in triangular shapes and used for packed lunches and traveling. The umeboshi in the center helps to keep them fresh longer. Use freshly cooked rice to form rice balls. Warm pressure-cooked rice shapes and holds the form easier than boiled or baked rice. Cool slightly before placing nori on rice balls as hot rice will crinkle the nori.

Learn to make rice balls with plain rice before attempting variations. Variations include: making smaller forms such as cylinders or walnut-sized balls; preparing a mixed rice such as azuki bean or rye berry with brown rice; mixing cooked rice with gomashio (sesame seed salt) or shiso powder to form rice balls; or covering formed rice balls with gomashio or roasted, chopped sunflower seeds or almonds.

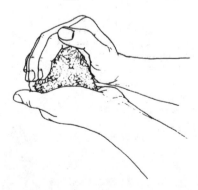

Noodles

Use – Noodles used in macrobiotic cooking are made from whole grains. These noodles, like whole cereal grains, can form the basis of a meal. Pastas are made from a variety of grains such as whole wheat, buckwheat, rice, corn, quinoa, and spelt. Wheat free noodles are available for those who are wheat sensitive.

Noodles and salt – Japanese noodles such as udon (wheat) and soba (buckwheat) often contain salt while American and European noodles usually do not. Check the package. If salted, boil in unsalted water. If unsalted, boil in salted water. When cooking dishes with salted noodles, reduce the indicated amount of salt.

Preparations – There are two basic ways to prepare noodles. The first method is to boil noodles, drain, and serve or mix with other ingredients. Use as a main course, in a salad or casserole, or serve in broth. Kids often like pastas prepared this way and served just as they are.

A second preparation method is to cook noodles together with additional ingredients. This way makes a "minestrone-type" soup or one-pot meal, uses fewer pans, and saves time. See the Soups and the Beans chapters for recipes that also include noodles.

Cooking time – Noodles require 7 to 15 minutes of boiling. They are done when they are tender and have a uniform color throughout. Cook noodles until tender, but still firm. If too soft, they may fall apart when serving or mixing into a dish. When cooking noodles into a dish, add during the last 10 to 15 minutes of cooking.

Noodles made with durum wheat hold up well to the boiling and stirring that is necessary for cooking noodles. When cooking noodles without wheat, use the shock method that follows on the next page; it helps to cook the pasta thoroughly while retaining its shape.

Serving – Cooked noodles can be served with broths, soups, sauces, or garnishes. Since noodles absorb flavor, more than the usual amount of seasoning is required. Always taste and adjust seasonings. Cooked noodles also can be used in salads, casseroles, and sea vegetable dishes.

To ease the serving of long spaghetti noodles, place noodles into a serving bowl with some care rather than heaping all together. Measure one serving at a time by hand and place into a serving bowl or platter with a small twist to maintain placement and presentation. It is easy to pick up one serving at a time without pulling out all the noodles.

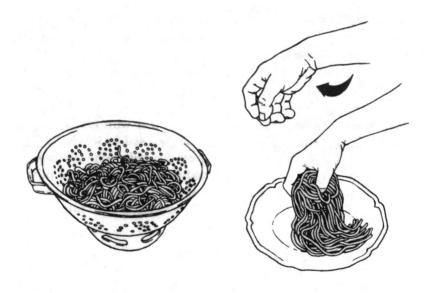

Boiled Noodles, Shock Method

Procedure – Bring water to a boil. Add sea salt if needed. Add noodles and stir to separate them. Bring to a rolling boil. Add ½ cup cold water and stir noodles. Bring to a rolling boil a second time. Immediately, add ½ cup cold water and stir noodles. Bring to a rolling boil a third time. Add ½ cup cold water and stir noodles. Bring to a rolling boil again.

Noodles are done when they are the same color inside and out. Drain. Rinse in cold water. Drain. Rinse and drain again, if needed, until noodles are cooled.

Noodles – Yield: 5 to 6 cups per 8 ounces noodles.

---

4 quarts of water for up to 16 ounces of noodles
¼ tsp sea salt for 4 quarts of water, for unsalted noodles

Comments – Shocking is the preferred method of cooking noodles that have reduced or no wheat. Buckwheat (soba), corn, and rice noodles are delicate. Shocking allows the noodles to cook thoroughly and gently. The cold water temporarily halts the cooking of the outside of the noodles so the inside of the noodles can catch up.

To shock: bring the noodles to a rolling boil, and add cold water. Repeat twice. Cold water is added a total of three times.

For the best flavor and balance, use salt in noodles. American- and European-style pastas usually are salt-free, so cook in salted water. Japanese noodles (soba and udon) usually contain salt. Cook in unsalted water. Check the packaging.

The cooking water can be saved for later use. Cool water to room temperature and refrigerate. Use within 2 to 3 days to cook other grains, soups, and breads.

Noodles—Menu suggestions

Procedure – Cook noodles with the shock method and serve as directed.

Soba, page 75
Kombu clear soup, page 124
Pan-fried perch, page 155, or pan-fried tofu, page 151
– Serve soba with perch or tofu and garnish with lemon
    wedge, scallions, nori matchsticks, page 134, and op-
    tional avocado and tomato wedges
Green vegetable dish of choice

Soba, page 75
Soba broth with tofu, page 123
Garnish: scallions and nori matchsticks, page 134
– Serve soba in soba broth with tofu and garnish
Grain burgers, page 251
Green vegetable dish of choice
Pickle of choice

Soba, page 75
Specialty dressing, page 167
Pan-fried tempeh, page 152
Garnish: scallions, cucumber, and avocado
– Serve soba with specialty dressing topped with pan-fried
    tempeh and garnish

Udon, page 75
Onion soup, page 111
– Serve udon in onion soup
Baked sweet potato chips, page 82
Choice of green salad

Udon, page 75
Caramelized onions, page 93
Garnish: roasted walnuts or almonds, pages 183-184
    (chopped) and parsley
– Serve udon with caramelized onions and garnish
Fish or other protein dish of choice

Corn pasta, page 75
Pesto, page 179
– Serve corn pasta with pesto
Azuki beans with onion, page 139
Leafy greens, page 103
Olive oil and umeboshi vinegar dressing, page 167

Corn pasta, page 75
Stir-fried vegetables, pages 88-89
Garnish: roasted dulse, page 134
– Serve corn pasta with stir-fried vegetables
Fish or other protein dish of choice

Spiral pasta, page 75
Blanched snow peas, page 100
Caramelized onions, page 93
Specialty dressing, page 167
Garnish: roasted almonds, pages 183-184
– Serve spiral pasta with snow peas, onions, specialty dress-
    ing, and garnish
Fish or other protein dish of choice

Comments – Other sauces good to serve on top of noodles include: tofu sauces; tahini sauces; clear sauces, espccially with steamed vegetables for low-fat meals; and tomato-based sauces, see page 93. See the Sauces and Condiments chapter for full preparation instructions.

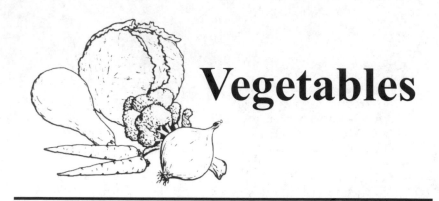

Vegetables

Use – Vegetables add color, flavor, and balance to the hearty dietary foundation of whole grains. They can be used at each meal, rotated with the season and for variety. Use as much of the vegetable as possible. Most vegetable skins are edible; even the skin of winter squash cooks tender. Cabbage hearts and broccoli stems are delicious, too. Any woody parts can be trimmed.

Cleaning – Clean vegetables to remove bad spots and dirt. Peel onions and waxed vegetables. Sort through greens to remove wilted and discolored leaves. If roots have embedded dirt, use the inside point of a knife to scrape off this dirt as shown in the illustration.

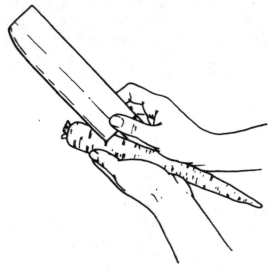

Washing – Wash vegetables after cleaning. Scrub roots with a vegetable brush. Immerse leafy greens and scallions individually in a basin of water. Don't take short cuts when washing vegetables. It may seem faster to rinse under the faucet, but it may not remove all the dirt.

Cutting – Learn and use various cutting styles. Cut vegetables into larger pieces when cooked alone than when cooked in combination. When vegetables are cooked together, use different, yet complementary, cuts so the dish is attractive. Cut vegetables in similar sizes for uniform cooking. Generally, cut young and tender vegetables into larger pieces than older vegetables. For cutting styles, see pages 43-55.

Cooking and timing – Overcooking can ruin some vegetables (broccoli and cauliflower become mushy), while undercooking can ruin others (butternut squash remains hard). Generally, green vegetables can be slightly undercooked, and orange/yellow vegetables can be slightly overcooked. The age of the vegetable affects the length of cooking. Younger vegetables are more tender than older vegetables and require shorter cooking times. The cutting style, too, affects the length of cooking. Smaller pieces cook faster than larger pieces.

Sea salt – Sea salt helps bring out the flavor of vegetables, especially the sweetness of onions, carrots, and squashes. For greens, sea salt is often omitted as it can make them bitter. For vegetables high in potassium such as cabbage or tomatoes and potatoes, sea salt is used to maintain an acceptable balance of sodium and potassium.

Potatoes, tomatoes, green peppers, and avocados – Many macrobiotic books recommend avoiding potatoes and tomatoes completely along with eggplant, green peppers, and avocados. Personally, we include them from time to time, especially on holidays or for guests. Thus, they are included in this book along with suggestions to help balance these foods.

Baked Vegetables, Whole

Procedure – Pierce vegetables with fork, knife, or ice pick so that there are air holes on top, every inch or so. Place vegetables on an oiled baking sheet. Bake 1 to 1½ hours at 350 degrees until vegetables are soft and a fork can be inserted easily.

> **Baked vegetables** – Use any combination, singly or mixed, of the following.
>
> ---
>
> butternut or acorn winter squash, small to medium
> sweet potatoes, medium to large
> potatoes, large, see page 79
> turnips, medium
> onions, large
>
> ---

Comments – It is easy to bake whole vegetables; however, not all vegetables can be baked. This method works best with vegetables that retain their shape such as root vegetables. To make the skin softer, lightly oil the vegetables before baking.

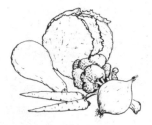

Baked Vegetables, Cut

Procedure – Place water to a depth of ½ inch in casserole dish. Mix vegetables with sea salt and add to dish. Cover. Bake 45 minutes to 1 hour at 350 degrees, or until tender.

Winter squash – Yield: 7 cups.

---

3 pounds winter squash, 1½-inch squares, 8 cups
⅛ tsp sea salt
water as needed

Carrots and onion – Yield: 4 cups.

---

1 medium onion, minced, 1½ cups
4 medium carrots, diced or shaved, 3 cups
⅛ tsp sea salt
water as needed

Sweet potatoes and parsnips – Yield: 7 cups.

---

1 medium onion, thick crescents, 1½ cups
3 medium sweet potatoes, "logs," 5 cups
2 medium parsnips, large matchsticks, 1½ cups
¼ tsp sea salt
water as needed

Comments – Bake vegetables for ease of preparation and to bring out their sweetness. While some vegetables such as butternut squash bake well when whole, others such as kabocha squash and carrots bake better when cut. Rutabagas, turnips, beets, whole onions, and leeks can be baked also.

Baked Vegetables, Oil Coated

Procedure – Mix vegetables, oil, and sea salt. Spread evenly on an oiled baking sheet. Bake 1 hour at 350 degrees or until tender.

Sweet potato chips or fries – Yield: 2½ cups.

> 2 medium sweet potatoes or yams, thin rounds or "logs,"
>   3 cups
> 2 Tbsp coconut oil, melted
> ¼ tsp sea salt

Parsnip chips – Yield: 2½ cups.

> 4 medium parsnips, thin diagonals, 3 cups
> 2 Tbsp coconut oil, melted
> ¼ tsp sea salt

French fries – See note regarding the use of potatoes on page 79. Yield: 5 cups.

> 6 medium red, yellow, or Russet potatoes, "logs," 6 cups
> 4 Tbsp coconut oil, melted
> ½ tsp sea salt

Comments – Sweet potatoes, parsnips, and potatoes, if used, bake well. Try other root vegetables singly or mixed. When cutting vegetables, try to make all cuts as uniform as possible. You can save time by making the cuts smaller and baking at 375 degrees for 45 minutes.

This procedure is useful for preparing French fries. Make your own at home for kids or for anyone needing transitional foods, and to avoid fast food restaurants. See pages 16-17 on the use of oil.

Layered Vegetables

Procedure – Heat oil in a pan. Sauté onion until transparent. Add water. Layer vegetables in the order listed. Sprinkle sea salt on top. Cover and bring to a boil. Simmer over low heat for time indicated.

Cabbage and carrots – Simmer 20 minutes. Yield: 5 cups.

½ tsp light sesame oil or olive oil
1 medium onion, thin crescents, 1½ cups
1 medium cabbage; 5 cups
    core, diced
    leaves, 1-inch squares
1 large carrot, large matchsticks, 1 cup
½ cup water
¼ tsp sea salt

Winter squash and carrots – Simmer 30 minutes. Yield: 7 cups.

½ tsp light sesame oil or olive oil
1 medium onion, thin crescents, 1½ cups
½ cup water
1 medium butternut squash, 2-inch squares, 6 cups
3 medium carrots, small chunks, 2 cups
½ tsp sea salt

Summer squash and green beans – Simmer 10 minutes. Yield: 5 cups.

½ tsp light sesame oil or olive oil
1 medium onion, thin crescents, 1½ cups
½ cup water
4 medium yellow squash, "paper cut," 4 cups
25 large green beans, 3-inch lengths, 2 cups
¼ tsp sea salt

Brussels sprouts, cauliflower, and carrots – Simmer 10 to 15 minutes. Yield: 7 cups.

½ tsp light sesame oil or olive oil
1 medium onion, thin crescents, 1½ cups
½ cup water
½ medium cauliflower, large flowerets, 3 cups
12 medium Brussels sprouts, whole, 3 cups, cut an "x" into the bottom of each Brussels sprout to help cook faster
4 medium carrots, large chunks, 3 cups
½ tsp sea salt

Comments – Layering is a simple way to cook 3 or 4 kinds of vegetables together. Onion is sautéed first to add flavor. Then the vegetables are layered from yin at the bottom to yang on the top. There are many possible combinations. Try using greens, leeks, corn cut off the cob, or unusual vegetables such as sunchokes.

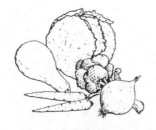

Layered Vegetables with Cornmeal

Procedure – Roast cornmeal in a dry pan until fragrant, 2 to 3 minutes, stirring constantly. Remove and set aside. Using the same pan, heat oil. Sauté onion until transparent. Add water. Layer vegetables in the order listed. Sprinkle cornmeal on top. Sprinkle sea salt on top of the cornmeal. Cover and bring to a boil. Simmer 30 minutes over low heat. Mix, cover, and let stand 5 minutes before serving. Cornmeal will absorb all the liquid.

Collard greens with cornmeal – Yield: 5 cups.

½ cup fine cornmeal
1 tsp light sesame oil or olive oil
1 medium onion, thin crescents, 1½ cups
1½ cups water
1 medium bunch collard greens;
    stems, thin rounds, 1 cup
    leaves, shredded, 8 cups
¼ tsp sea salt

Green peppers with cornmeal – See page 79. Yield: 3 cups.

½ cup fine cornmeal
1 tsp light sesame oil or olive oil
1 medium onion, thin crescents, 1½ cups
1½ cups water
4 medium green bell peppers, thin crescents, 3 cups
¼ tsp sea salt

Comments – Layer vegetables with cornmeal to produce a hearty vegetable dish. It is a delicious way to serve greens. Try other combinations, layering from yin to yang, such as onion, cabbage, turnip, and carrot.

Pressure-Cooked Vegetables

Procedure – Place vegetables, water, and sea salt in a pressure cooker. Bring to full pressure as per pressure cooker instructions. Cook for the time indicated. Bring pressure down immediately by running cold water over the top of the cooker.

Butternut squash and onions – Pressure cook 10 minutes. Yield: 12 cups.

> 3 large onions, halved
> 1 large butternut squash, 3 pounds, 3-inch squares
> ½ cup water
> ¼ tsp sea salt

Turnips, rutabagas, and carrots – Use an equal amount of turnip and rutabaga. Peel rutabaga if waxed. Pressure cook 8 minutes. Yield: 6 cups.

> 1 large onion, quartered
> 2 large turnips, 8 pieces
> 2 large rutabagas, turnip-size, 8 pieces
> 2 large carrots, chunks
> ½ cup water
> ¼ tsp sea salt

Corn on the cob – Pressure cook 3 to 4 minutes. Yield: 4 ears of corn.

> 4 ears corn
> ½ cup water
> pinch sea salt

Combinations – Each of the following vegetables take 2 minutes to pressure cook. Use singly or mix as you wish. Add ½ cup water to the pressure cooker. Use ⅛ tsp sea salt per 4 cups vegetables.

---

green beans, whole
broccoli, flowerets
cauliflower, flowerets
greens, shredded
cabbage, shredded
Brussels sprouts, whole
yellow and zucchini squash, ½-inch rounds
onion, thin crescents

Comments – Pressure cooking vegetables saves time, especially for hearty root vegetables or when cooking vegetables for many people. Cut vegetables into smaller pieces for faster cooking, similar-sized pieces when combining vegetables, and time carefully for best results. Most vegetables can be pressure cooked.

Vegetables that are sautéed can also be pressure cooked. Celery and parsnips, page 89, and Burdock and carrots, page 94, are delicious when prepared this way. Sauté in pressure cooker, add water and soy sauce as directed, bring to full pressure, and cook for one-third of the recommended simmering time—5 minutes for celery and parsnips, 10 minutes for burdock and carrots.

For information on using a pressure cooker, see pages 38-41.

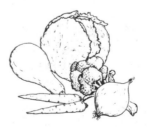

Sautéed and Stir-Fried Vegetables

Procedure – Heat oil in a pan over medium to medium-high heat. Sauté onion until transparent. Add the first vegetable listed and sauté briefly. Add remaining vegetables, one kind at a time, in the order listed. Sauté and stir each kind briefly before adding the next one. Add sea salt and water. Cover and bring to a boil. Turn heat to low and simmer 5 to 7 minutes for crisp vegetables, or up to 20 minutes for more tender vegetables. Add soy sauce if using. If using a wok, see comments.

Butternut squash and kale – Simmer 15 minutes. Yield: 6½ cups.

---

1 tsp light sesame oil or olive oil
1 medium onion, thin crescents, 1½ cups
1 medium butternut squash, ½-inch squares, 6 cups
1 medium bunch kale;
    stems, thin diagonals, ½ cup
    leaves, 1-inch squares, 6 cups
¼ tsp sea salt
½ cup water
½ tsp soy sauce, optional

Yellow squash, cabbage, and carrots – Simmer 7 minutes. Yield: 5 cups.

---

1 tsp light sesame oil or olive oil
1 medium onion, thin crescents, 1½ cups
1 medium carrot, thin matchsticks, ¾ cup
3 medium yellow squash, "paper cut," 3 cups
½ small cabbage, core removed, shredded, 3 cups
½ cup water
¼ tsp sea salt
½ tsp soy sauce, optional

Snow peas and carrots and tofu – Marinate tofu in soy sauce while sautéing vegetables. Drain and reserve soy sauce. Add tofu after the last vegetable is sautéed. Cover and simmer together 7 minutes over low heat. Use reserved soy sauce to season. Yield: 4½ cups.

½ pound tofu, ½-inch cubes, 2 cups
1 Tbsp soy sauce
1 tsp light sesame oil or olive oil
1 medium onion, thin crescents, 1½ cups
3 medium carrots, large matchsticks, 2 cups
25 whole medium snow peas, 1 cup
¼ tsp sea salt
½ cup water

Broccoli – Simmer 5 minutes. Yield: 5 cups.

½ tsp light sesame oil or olive oil
1 medium onion, thin crescents, 1½ cups
1 medium bunch broccoli; 6 cups
    stems, thin diagonals
    2½-inch long flowerets, ½-inch thick at stem
¼ tsp sea salt
½ cup water

Celery and parsnips – Onion is not used in this recipe. Simmer 15 minutes. Yield: 5 cups.

½ tsp light sesame oil or olive oil
4 medium stalks celery, thin diagonals, 3 cups
4 medium parsnips, large matchsticks, 3 cups
¼ tsp sea salt
½ cup water

Comments – Sautéing and stir-frying are similar cooking methods. Both cook vegetables in minimal oil, the difference being in length of cooking and amount of stirring. Shorter times produce crisp vegetables that retain their bright colors. Longer times produce more tender vegetables.

Cook vegetables in oil and stir with each addition; onions first, then remaining vegetables in yang to yin order. After all the vegetables are added, simmer until tender. Use as many vegetables as desired; three kinds are visually appealing. Sauté and stir-fry vegetables in a wok or a regular pan and serve as a main dish, side dish, or over rice or pasta.

If using a wok, sauté the first vegetable in the middle of the pan where the heat is concentrated. Sauté briefly, then push the sautéed vegetables to the side of the wok and add the next vegetable to the middle of the wok over the heat. Sauté in the middle briefly, then mix with the already sautéed vegetables. Repeat with remaining vegetables. Add water and sea salt. Cover and bring to a boil. Simmer until tender.

Use ginger for variety and flavor. Add 2 to 3 teaspoons of freshly minced ginger to the oil and sauté very briefly, until fragrant. Add onion and continue with any of the combinations listed.

Make sauce for another variation. Dilute 2 teaspoons arrowroot or 1 teaspoon kuzu powder with ½ teaspoon soy sauce, ¼ cup cold water, and a dash of toasted sesame oil if desired. Add to the vegetables after they have simmered. Gently mix and cook until sauce becomes thick and transparent, about 15 seconds.

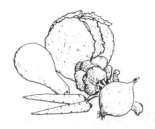

Sautéed Vegetables with Miso

Procedure – Heat oil in a pan. Sauté vegetables with sea salt, if used, until color changes, 1 to 2 minutes. Add water, if used. Cover and bring to a boil. Simmer over low heat until tender, 10 to 15 minutes. Add miso in small pats on top of the vegetables. Cover and simmer 5 minutes to soften miso. Stir miso into the vegetables.

Scallion miso – Sauté greens, then whites. Yield: 1 cup.

> 2 tsp light sesame oil or olive oil
> 2 bunches scallion, thin rounds, 3 cups
> 4 tsp soybean, barley, and/or rice miso

Onion miso – Yield: 3 cups.

> 2 tsp light sesame oil or olive oil
> 4 medium onions, thin crescents, 6 cups
> ¼ tsp sea salt
> 2 Tbsp water
> 3 to 4 tsp soybean, barley, and/or rice miso

Green pepper miso – See page 79. Yield: 2 cups.

> 2 tsp light sesame oil or olive oil
> 4 medium green peppers, thin crescents, 3 cups
> ¼ tsp sea salt
> 4 tsp soybean, barley, and/or rice miso

Comments – Vegetables cooked with miso make an appetizing side dish or spread—2 to 3 tablespoons per serving. Scallions will cook in their own juice without sea salt, but onions and green peppers need sea salt to draw out their juice. These are classic recipes, but also try leeks, carrots, or "carrot tops" (the leafy green part, discard stem) with miso, or using less or a lighter miso to make a milder vegetable dish.

Sautéed Vegetables without Water

Procedure – Heat oil in a pan. Sauté onion with a pinch of sea salt until transparent. Add vegetables and the rest of the sea salt and sauté 1 to 2 minutes. Stir constantly. Cover. Simmer over low heat for the time indicated, or until tender, stirring once or twice.

Cabbage – Simmer 15 to 20 minutes. Yield: 3 cups.

1 tsp light sesame oil or olive oil
1 medium onion, thin crescents, 1½ cups
½ medium cabbage; 5 cups
    core, finely minced
    leaves, 1-inch squares
½ tsp sea salt

Mustard greens – Simmer 10 to 15 minutes. Yield: 3½ cups.

1 tsp light sesame oil or olive oil
1 medium onion, thin crescents, 1½ cups
1 medium bunch mustard greens; 8 cups
    stems, finely minced
    leaves, shredded
¼ tsp sea salt

Summer squash – Simmer 20 to 25 minutes. Yield: 5 cups.

1 tsp light sesame oil or olive oil
1 medium onion, thin crescents, 1½ cups
4 medium yellow squash, "paper cut," 4 cups
4 medium zucchini, "paper cut," 4 cups
½ tsp sea salt

Caramelized onions or buttery onion sauce – Simmer 20 to 25 minutes. To caramelize, leave cover off. For soft buttery onions, use cover. Yield: 1½ cups.

---

2 Tbsp light sesame oil or olive oil
2 medium onions, thin crescents, 3 cups
½ tsp sea salt

Watercress – Omit sea salt. Simmer 5 minutes. Add soy sauce at the end of cooking. Yield: 1½ cups.

½ tsp light sesame oil or olive oil
1 bunch watercress, finely sliced, 4 cups
⅛ tsp soy sauce

Chinese cabbage and carrots – Simmer 10 to 15 minutes. Yield: 4 cups.

---

1 tsp light sesame oil or olive oil
½ large Chinese cabbage; 6 cups
   core, finely minced
   leaves, 1-inch squares
1 medium carrot, thin matchsticks, ¾ cup
¼ tsp sea salt

Comments – Sautéing without water is a method used specifically with vegetables that contain enough water that they will simmer in their own juices when sprinkled with sea salt. Sea salt draws out water for listed vegetables, plus others such as daikon radish, scallions, green peppers, and okra. Vegetables without excess water such as carrots can be used if added to watery vegetables, such as carrots with mustard greens. For extra flavor, season with soy sauce at the end of cooking.

This way of cooking works well with tomatoes, if you wish to use them, see page 79. Sauté in oil with sea salt to help balance the yin quality of tomatoes. For tomato sauce, use onion, garlic, tomato, sea salt, and herbs such as basil and oregano.

Sautéed Vegetables with Soy Sauce

Procedure – Heat oil in a pan. Sauté vegetables with sea salt, in the order listed, until fragrant, 1 to 2 minutes. Add water and soy sauce. Cover and bring to a boil. Simmer 25 minutes over low heat. Uncover and cook to evaporate remaining water.

Carrots – Yield: 3 cups.

1 tsp light sesame oil or olive oil
1 medium onion, thin crescents, 1½ cups
4 medium carrots, large matchsticks, 3 cups
⅛ tsp sea salt
½ cup water
1 Tbsp soy sauce

Burdock and carrots (kinpira) – Cut the burdock and carrots in the same style, either thin matchsticks or small shavings, with the burdock pieces smaller than the carrot pieces. To cook burdock: sauté burdock with a dash of sea salt for 1 minute, with the cover on the pan. Remove cover, stir in another dash of sea salt, replace the cover and sauté another minute. Repeat for a third time. Burdock should smell fragrant. Then add carrots, the rest of the sea salt, and proceed as above. Yield: 3 cups.

2 to 3 Tbsp light sesame oil
2 small burdock roots, thin matchsticks or shavings,
    1½ cups
4 medium carrots, thin matchsticks or shavings, 3 cups
¼ tsp salt
¾ cup water
1 Tbsp soy sauce

Rutabagas – Peel rutabagas if waxed. Yield: 3 cups.

---

1 tsp light sesame oil
1 medium onion, minced, 1½ cups
3 medium rutabagas, diced, 3 cups
⅛ tsp sea salt
½ cup water
1 Tbsp soy sauce

Comments – Sautéing with soy sauce is especially recommended for root vegetables as soy sauce creates a flavorful and hearty dish. This method is a thorough and delicious way to cook burdock taught to me by my Japanese teacher, Cornellia Aihara. Vary by cooking burdock by itself and serving with a sprinkling of roasted sesame seeds or gomashio. Or, cook with soaked shiitake mushrooms.

Use this method of sautéing burdock for other dishes. Sautéed burdock can be added to miso soup, sea vegetable dishes, or grain and vegetable dishes.

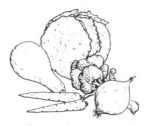

Water-"Sautéed" Vegetables

Procedure – Add water to pan and heat to a boil. Without covering pan, add vegetables and sea salt. Stir constantly until tender.

Scallions – Yield: about ¾ cup.

2 to 3 Tbsp water
1 bunch scallions, thin rounds, 1½ cups
pinch of sea salt

Chinese cabbage – Yield: 1 cup.

2 to 3 Tbsp water
3 leaves Chinese Cabbage, shredded, 2 cups
pinch of sea salt

Comments – Water-sautéed vegetables is a method of preparing vegetables where ¼ inch of water is brought to a boil and vegetables are "sautéed" by constantly stirring. The vegetables are cooked quickly. Water sautéing is a useful procedure when cooking for one or two people and for those wanting to avoid oil and/or raw food. Vegetables retain their crunchiness. Many kinds of vegetables can be prepared in this manner, singly or in combination, as long as cuts are small and quantity is minimal. Most nutritive value remains due to the short cooking time.

Simmered Vegetables, Salted Water

Procedure – Bring water to a boil. Add sea salt. Add vegetables. Cover and bring to a boil. Simmer for the time indicated over low heat.

Broccoli – Simmer stems 1 minute, then add flowerets and simmer 5 to 7 minutes. Yield: 4 cups.

½ cup water
¼ tsp sea salt
1 medium bunch broccoli; 6 cups
   stems, "logs"
   3-inch long flowerets, ½-inch thick at stem

Corn on the cob – Simmer 7 to 10 minutes. Yield: 4 pieces.

½ cup water
⅛ tsp sea salt
2 large ears of corn, broken or cut into 4-inch pieces

Beets – Simmer 20 to 30 minutes. Yield: 4 cups.

½ cup water
¼ tsp sea salt
6 medium beets, quarter rounds, 4½ cups

Comments – Water boils at 212 degrees. Adding salt raises the boiling point of water and thus vegetables cook with higher heat. Green beans and broccoli are delicious. When using this method, take care to bring water to a complete boil before adding sea salt and vegetables.

A variation of this method is to use a vegetable steamer, simply steaming vegetables over gently boiling salted water until tender. This way is appropriate for anyone on a reduced sodium diet.

Simmered Vegetables

Procedure – Place water in a pan. Layer vegetables in the order listed. Sprinkle sea salt on top. Cover and bring to a boil. Simmer for the time indicated over low heat.

Carrots – Simmer 20 to 30 minutes. Yield: 6 cups.

½ cup water
6 large carrots, big chunks or "logs," 6 cups
¼ tsp sea salt

Green beans – Simmer 7 to 10 minutes. Yield: 4 cups.

½ cup water
1 pound green beans, 2-inch lengths, 4½ cups
¼ tsp sea salt

Sweet potatoes – Simmer 30 minutes to 2 hours—the longer the cooking time, the more flavorful. Yield: 5 to 6 cups.

1 to 1½ cups water
4 large sweet potatoes, large matchsticks or chunks, 10
    cups
½ tsp sea salt

Green beans, corn, and red onions – Simmer 10 minutes. Yield: 3½ cups.

½ cup water
1 medium red onion, minced, 1½ cups
25 medium green beans, ½-inch rounds, 2 cups
2 medium ears of corn, cut off the cob, 2 cups
¼ tsp sea salt

Cabbage – Simmer 10 minutes. Yield: 3 cups.

½ cup water
½ medium cabbage, core removed, shredded, 5 cups
¼ tsp sea salt

Winter squash – Simmer 30 minutes. Yield: 8 cups.

1 cup water
1 large butternut or other squash, 2-inch squares, 10 cups
¼ tsp sea salt

Spaghetti squash – Simmer 20 to 25 minutes. Serve with oil and soy sauce dressing, page 170. Yield: 6 cups.

1 cup water
1 spaghetti squash, 3 pounds, quartered
¼ tsp sea salt

Comments – This procedure is a simple, easy way to cook vegetables. Simmering with sea salt on top cooks the sea salt into the vegetables and brings out the sweet flavor. Most vegetables can be simmered in this way, with the exception of leafy greens, which can become bitter. For leafy greens, see page 103.

Cook vegetables singly or in combination. When using more than one vegetable, layer from yin at the bottom to yang at the top. The size of the cuts affects the flavor and the amount of cooking time. The smaller the cuts, the faster the vegetables cook. For winter squashes and sweet potatoes, large cuts and long cooking times bring out more flavor.

Add nut or seed butter to cooked vegetables to make a sauce-like dish. Dilute 2 tablespoons tahini in ¼ cup cooking water and add 1 teaspoon soy sauce. Add to 4 cups cooked vegetables when tender, especially green beans or vegetable combinations. Cook until thick, 1 to 2 minutes, stirring constantly.

Boiled Vegetables, Whole Vegetables

Procedure – Bring water to a boil in a large pan over high heat. Add sea salt. Cook vegetables in the order listed, one kind at a time. Bring to a boil without covering pan. Boil until vegetables are cooked to desired texture, crisp or tender. Remove with a slotted spoon or strainer. Drain in colander. Separate pieces so they cool. Repeat with each kind of vegetable. Cool completely. Cut. Gently mix with dressing, add toppings, or serve as dipping vegetables.

Green beans with almonds – Simmer 4 minutes for crisp green beans—up to 8 minutes for more tender. Yield: 2 cups.

> 4 cups water
> ⅛ tsp sea salt
> 25 large green beans, whole, 2 cups; cut into 2-inch
>   lengths when cool
> Dressing: Nut butter dressing; use almond butter, soy
>   sauce, brown rice vinegar, and water, page 166;
> or, Topping: Roasted almonds, ½ cup, with soy sauce,
>   pages 183-184

Snow peas – Useful as a garnish. Simmer 2 to 3 minutes. After boiling, briefly dip in cold water to halt cooking and retain color. Yield: 1 cup.

> 4 cups water
> pinch of sea salt
> 25 snow peas, about ¼ pound, trimmed but left whole,
>   1 cup

Salad vegetables and dips – For cauliflower and broccoli, stand upright, stem closest to bottom of pan. Boil 4 to 5 minutes until a toothpick can be inserted into stem, then turn and boil flower side down another 30 seconds. Cook cauliflower first to retain color. Yield: 8 cups.

---

6 cups water
¼ tsp sea salt
1 small cauliflower; leave whole but remove hard bottom stem; separate into flowerets after cooking
1 small bunch broccoli; cut each stalk 3 inches below flower; separate into flowerets after cooking
3 medium carrots, halved; cut into "logs" after cooking
Dipping sauce: Tofu and tahini sauce, page 182;
    or, Walnut sauce with soy sauce, page 179;
    or, Nut butter sauce, page 178

Comments – This book includes three listings for boiled vegetables: whole, cut, and leafy vegetables. Vegetables boiled without a cover keep their bright color, and stay crisp if removed immediately or when the water returns to a boil. After cooking, drain and separate pieces to cool completely. Vegetables can be submerged in cool water if needed to stop the cooking. Cut when cool.

Whole vegetables require longer boiling time than cut vegetables and retain more flavor. When boiling whole vegetables, cook one kind of vegetable at a time for uniform tenderness. When cooking more than one kind, cook in order of "color" to preserve brightness. For example, cauliflower would absorb other colors, so cook it first.

Use the cooking water to boil noodles or season with soy sauce and serve as a clear soup. Cooking water also can be saved and used as stock for vegetable soups.

Boiled vegetables can be used in salads if crisp or as a vegetable dish if tender. The procedure lends itself to experimenting. Quickly boiled green beans or yellow squash can be added to a raw lettuce salad. Tender but firm parsnips can be cooked whole and then cut for use with dips.

Boiled Vegetables, Cut Vegetables

Procedure – Bring water to a boil in a large pan over high heat. Add sea salt. Cook any desired number of vegetables, one kind at a time, starting with light-colored vegetables first. Bring to a boil without covering pan. For crisp vegetables cut in thin pieces and remove when water returns to a rolling boil—within 10 seconds. For tender vegetables, boil each kind up to 5 minutes, then remove. Drain and spread thinly to cool. Repeat with each kind of vegetable. Cool completely. Serve separately or gently mix all vegetables together with or without dressing.

Cabbage, carrot, and celery "cooked salad" – Yield: 5½ cups.

6 cups water
¼ tsp sea salt
1 small cabbage, core removed, shredded, 5 cups
2 medium celery stalks, thin diagonals, 1½ cups
1 medium carrot, thin matchsticks, ¾ cup
Dressing: Soy sauce dressing, use lemon juice, page 166;
    or, Umeboshi and nut butter dressing, use 3 plums
       and 2 Tbsp lemon juice, page 169;
    or, Onion and lemon dressing, page 168

These vegetables are delicious cooked with this procedure:

onions, crescents
daikon radish, thin rounds or matchsticks
tender yellow summer squash, thin rounds
turnips, thin quarter rounds
broccoli flowerets
Chinese cabbage, shredded

Comments – See comments under Boiled Vegetables, Whole Vegetables, page 100.

Boiled Vegetables, Leafy Greens

Procedure – Bring water to a boil in a large pan over high heat. Add vegetables and return to a boil without covering pan. Boil briefly, 1 to 2 minutes, or up to 5 minutes if thick.

For whole greens, stand up in pan, so that the stems or hard parts are standing on the bottom. Immerse leafy parts when stems wilt, after about 1 minute of boiling.

Boil until done then remove to colander and spread to cool. When cool, squeeze gently to remove excess water. For whole greens, cut into 1-inch pieces. Gently mix with dressing.

Kale – Yield: 4 cups.

8 cups water
1 medium bunch kale, remove hard stems, cut leaves
　　into 1-inch squares, 8 cups
Dressing: Olive oil and umeboshi vinegar dressing, page 167

Mustard greens – Yield: 3 cups.

8 cups water
1 medium bunch mustard greens, whole leaves, 8 cups
Dressing: 2 to 3 Tbsp Sesame seed salt, page 186

Comments – This is a preferred method of preparing leafy vegetables such as kale, collards, mustard greens, baby bok choy, turnip greens, and radish greens. Some greens become bitter when steamed or sautéed. Boiling removes this bitterness. Salt also can make greens bitter so it is not used in the water. Greens can be boiled whole, for more flavor, or cut into strips or squares, to shorten cooking time. Boil quickly for crisp greens or longer for tougher greens. Dress with umeboshi vinegar, brown rice vinegar, or lemon juice. Oil and lemon dressing, page 170, is delicious. For variety, sauté greens (after boiling) in olive oil with garlic. Season with soy sauce and brown rice vinegar.

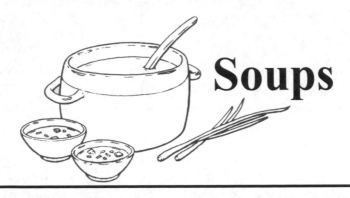

Soups

Cooking – Soups start a meal and offer variety and nutrition to a grain-based diet. From simple to fancy, soups soften and relax. There are two basic ways to make soup: boil all the ingredients together until tender, or sauté all or some of the ingredients first and then boil until tender. Soups with sautéed ingredients are generally more flavorful. Boiled soups save time as they require only one pan and can be made in minutes, as with Instant Vegetable Soups, page 106.

Vegetables – Cut different vegetables into similar-sized pieces so the cooking time is the same. Larger cuts require longer cooking times; smaller and finer cuts cook faster. Vary the cuts for a pleasing appearance, using big cuts for stews and bite-sized cuts for other soups. Older vegetables cook well into soup; longer cooking times make them tender. If you are in a hurry, use young vegetables because they cook more quickly. For most soups, use the same amount of water as cut vegetables, such as 2 cups of water per 2 cups of cut vegetables.

Pressure cooking – Many soups can be pressure cooked to save time. Follow the general pressure-cooking hints such as filling the cooker no more than two-thirds full and avoiding foods such as rolled oats, noodles, flour, tofu, dumplings, or wakame leaves that may clog the cooker. Follow the soup-making procedure to the "bring to a boil" stage. At that point, bring to full pressure. Pressure cook for one-third of the indicated time; for example, if the recipe calls for simmering 30 minutes, pressure cook for 10 minutes. If using foods that may clog the cooker, you may pressure cook the other ingredients and then simmer the dish after adding foods that should not be pressure cooked. For information on using a pressure cooker, see pages 38-41.

Stocks – A soup stock can be used in any soup in place of water for added flavor and nutrition. Kombu stock, page 124, can be used if desired. Vegetable stock can be made from vegetable scraps. Use 4 cups of clean unblemished vegetable scraps and cover with 8 cups water. Bring to a boil and simmer 30 minutes to 1 hour. Strain and remove scraps.

Seasoning – Miso and soy sauce are used most often to flavor soups in macrobiotic cooking. Miso and soy sauce are fermented products and are best when heated through but not boiled so that the beneficial bacteria are kept alive. Sometimes miso or soy sauce is cooked into a dish as in stews or condiments, but generally, for soups, it is added at the end of cooking and not boiled. Different kinds of miso can be used separately or mixed to season soup. Dark barley miso, aged about two years or more, is a good choice for daily miso soup.

If making soup for more than one meal, season only the portion to be served. Ladle desired amount into another pan and season, or season the individual bowls. Season soup to taste with miso or soy sauce. If soup is cooked with salt, it will need less seasoning.

To season: Dilute miso with ¼ cup or less hot broth, then mix miso with soup. For soy sauce, add directly to soup. Here are general proportions:

Soups with salt			Soups without salt		
amount	soy sauce	miso	amount	soy sauce	miso
1 cup	1 tsp	½ tsp	1 cup	1½ tsp	¾ tsp
2 cups	2 tsp	1 tsp	2 cups	1 Tbsp	1½ tsp
4 cups	4 tsp	2 tsp	4 cup	2 Tbsp	1 Tbsp

Instant Vegetable Soups

Procedure – Bring water to a boil. Add ingredients. Bring to a rolling boil. Remove from heat and add soy sauce or miso.

Instant orange soup – Yield: 5½ cups.

4 cups water
½ pound tofu, ½-inch cubes, 2 cups
1 small carrot, grated, ½ cup
3 medium scallions, thin rounds, ¾ cup
3 Tbsp soy sauce or 1½ Tbsp miso, see page 105

Instant white, green, and black soup – Yield: 5 cups.

4 cups water
1 cup grated daikon radish
1 cup watercress, minced
3 Tbsp soy sauce or 1½ Tbsp miso, see page 105
Garnish: 1 sheet nori, roasted and torn into squares, page 134

Wake-me-up instant soup – Inspired by Bob and Kathy Ligon. Yield: 1 cup.

1 cup water
1 tsp fresh ginger juice
1 clove garlic, crushed, 1 tsp
1 scallion, thin rounds, ¼ cup
½ tsp toasted sesame oil
1 tsp dark miso

Comments – Soups can be made instantly when using tofu, scallions, dulse, nori, couscous, finely grated vegetables, or leftovers. Kombu soups, pages 123-124, cook quickly and use many of the same ingredients.

Stews

Procedure – Measure water into a pan. Place kombu, if used, at the bottom. Layer vegetables from bottom to top in the order listed. Sprinkle sea salt on top. Cover and bring to a boil. Simmer 20 to 30 minutes over low heat until tender. Add soy sauce. Simmer another 5 minutes to cook soy sauce into the vegetables.

New England-style vegetable stew – Yield: 10 to 12 cups.

4 cups water
4 medium red potatoes, halved, 4 cups, see page 79
1 small cabbage, 8 crescents, 5 cups
4 medium onions, quartered, 4 cups
4 medium carrots, large chunks, 4 cups
½ tsp sea salt
2 Tbsp soy sauce, optional

Japanese-style vegetable stew, with kombu knots – Soak 4, six-inch pieces of kombu in 4 cups of water until pliable, 10 to 15 minutes. Slit each piece lengthwise into 1-inch wide strips. Tie each strip into a knot. Peel rutabagas if waxed. Yield: 14 cups.

4 cups kombu soaking water
16 kombu knots
4 medium onions, quartered, 4 cups
4 medium rutabagas (turnip sized), quartered, 4 cups
1 medium daikon radish, 1½-inch rounds, 4 cups
4 medium carrots, large chunks, 4 cups
½ tsp sea salt
2 Tbsp soy sauce

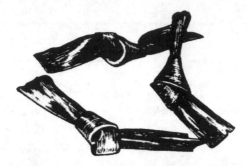

Comments – A stew is both a vegetable dish and a soup. The vegetables can be served on a plate if desired, while the broth is served in a bowl. The vegetables are often root vegetables cut into large pieces. Layer vegetables from yin at the bottom to yang at the top. Kombu knots cook tender and are a pretty addition. Try other root vegetables in stews such as turnips, parsnips, or burdock. Stews pressure cook well, see page 104.

Boiled Vegetable Soups

Procedure – Layer vegetables from bottom to top in the order listed. Add cold water. Sprinkle sea salt on top. Cover and bring to a boil. Simmer over low heat for the time indicated. Season with miso or soy sauce, page 105.

Kitchen soup – Simmer 30 minutes. Yield: 11 cups.

---

   1 large celery stalk, thin quarter rounds, ¾ cup
   1 small cabbage; 5 cups
      core, finely minced
      leaves, shredded
   1 medium onion, minced, 1½ cups
   1 medium carrot, thin quarter rounds, ¾ cup
   8 cups water
   ¼ tsp sea salt
   4 Tbsp soy sauce or 2 Tbsp miso

One-pot meal – Simmer vegetables 15 minutes. Add noodles and simmer 7 to 10 minutes. Add tofu and simmer 5
minutes. Season. Yield: 14 cups.

> 1 small butternut squash, 1-inch squares, 4 cups
> 1 large onion, thin crescents, 2 cups
> 1 large carrot, shaved, 1 cup
> 10 cups water
> ½ tsp sea salt
> 1 cup whole wheat ribbon noodles
> ½ pound tofu, ½-inch cubes, 2 cups
> 5 Tbsp soy sauce

Quick soup – Simmer 5 to 7 minutes. Garnish with scallions
and nori when serving soup. Yield: 6 cups.

> 3 Chinese cabbage leaves, shredded, 2 cups
> 2 yellow squash, thin quarter rounds, 2 cups
> 4 cups water
> ⅛ tsp sea salt
> 2 Tbsp soy sauce or 1 Tbsp miso
> Garnish: 1 medium scallion, thin rounds, ¼ cup
>   1 sheet nori, matchsticks, page 134

Comments – Many different soups can be made from this general procedure. Just layer vegetables from yin vegctables at the bottom to yang
vegetables at the top. Boil until tender, adding noodles, tofu, dumplings,
or garnishes as desired. Soup can be made quickly from young, finely
cut vegetables. Other combinations include: green beans, Chinese cabbage, and tofu as a quick soup; yellow squash, carrots, and noodles
garnished with scallions; and broccoli and fresh corn with dumplings.

Boiled Vegetable Soups, Creamy

Procedure – Layer vegetables from bottom to top in the order listed. Include any herbs or spices as desired. Add cold water. Sprinkle sea salt on top. Cover and bring to a boil. Simmer for the time indicated over low heat. Whisk nut or seed butter with arrowroot, soy sauce or miso, and rice milk. Add to soup. Stir to heat through and thicken but do not boil.

Creamy cauliflower soup with dumplings – Simmer vegetables for 15 minutes. Add dumplings and simmer 5 minutes. Season. Yield: 8½ cups.

4 to 5 large shallots, minced, ½ cup
1 medium cauliflower; 6 cups
   core, finely minced
   2-inch long flowerets, ½-inch thick at stem
minced garlic, ground black pepper, optional
5 cups water
¼ tsp sea salt
35 brown rice or whole wheat dumplings, page 212
4 Tbsp tahini
2 Tbsp arrowroot powder
2 Tbsp light miso
1 cup rice milk

Creamy macaroni soup – Simmer vegetables for 5 minutes. Add macaroni and simmer 7 to 10 minutes. Season. Yield: 8 cups.

1 medium onion, minced, 1½ cups
1 cup fresh green peas
1 ear fresh corn, cut off the cob, 1 cup
1 medium carrot, thin flowers, ¾ cup
minced garlic, curry powder, dill weed, optional
6 cups water
¼ tsp sea salt

> 1 cup whole wheat elbow macaroni
> 4 Tbsp tahini or almond butter
> 2 Tbsp arrowroot powder
> 3 Tbsp soy sauce
> 1 cup rice milk

Comments – Creamy boiled soup is a variation on the basic boiled soup. Diluted nut or seed butter is added to make it creamy. Try onion, broccoli, and noodle cream soup; or cream of carrot soup garnished with parsley.

Sautéed Vegetable Soups

Procedure – Heat water in a kettle. Heat oil in a pan and sauté onion with a pinch of sea salt until transparent, or sauté leek greens until bright green. Add vegetables in the order listed, one kind at a time. Sauté each kind for 1 to 2 minutes. Add boiling water and any spices used. Sprinkle remaining sea salt on top. Cover and bring to a boil. Simmer for the time indicated over low heat. Add soy sauce or miso, see seasoning, page 105.

> **Onion soup** – Sauté onions for 5 minutes for increased flavor. Simmer soup 30 to 35 minutes. Serve over cooked noodles or with croutons, page 258. Yield: 10 cups.

> > 2 tsp light sesame oil or olive oil
> > 5 medium onions, thin crescents, 7½ cups
> > ground black pepper, optional
> > 8 cups boiling water
> > ½ tsp sea salt
> > 4 Tbsp soy sauce or 2 Tbsp miso

Broccoli and tofu soup with dumplings – Sauté onion and then broccoli stems. Add water and simmer 10 minutes. Add flowerets, tofu, and dumplings and simmer 5 to 7 minutes. Season. Yield: 8 cups.

---

   1 tsp light sesame oil or olive oil
   1 medium onion, thin crescents, 1½ cups
   1 medium bunch broccoli; 6 cups
      stems, thin quarter rounds
      2-inch long broccoli flowerets, ½-inch thick at stem
   6 cups boiling water
   ¼ tsp sea salt
   35 brown rice or whole wheat dumplings, page 212
   ¼ pound tofu, ½-inch cubes, 1 cup
   ¼ cup soy sauce

Leek and squash soup – Wash leeks well before cutting. Simmer 30 minutes. Yield: 8½ cups.

   ½ tsp light sesame oil or olive oil
   1 large leek; 1½ cups
      greens, thin rounds
      whites, thin rounds
   1 small butternut squash, ½-inch squares, 4 cups
   6 cups boiling water
   ½ tsp sea salt
   3 Tbsp soy sauce

Comments – Many different soups can be made from this general procedure. Just sauté the vegetables, add water and sea salt, and simmer until tender, adding noodles, tofu, dumplings, or garnishes as desired. For other combinations, try onion, green beans, yellow squash, and carrots; leek, celery, and daikon; or winter squash and dumplings garnished with scallions and nori. All sautéed soups in this chapter are variations of this basic procedure.

Sautéed Vegetable Soups, Puréed

Procedure – Heat water in a kettle. Heat oil in a pan and sauté onion with a pinch of sea salt until transparent. Add vegetables in the order listed, one kind at time. Sauté each kind for 1 to 2 minutes. Add boiling water and spices if used. Sprinkle remaining sea salt on top. Cover and bring to a boil. Simmer 30 minutes over low heat. Purée in a blender or food mill, mash with a masher, or press through a sieve. Return to pan and bring to a boil. Add soy sauce, see page 105.

Golden soup – Yield: 14 cups.

1 tsp light sesame oil or olive oil
1 large onion, minced, 2 cups
1 large butternut squash, 1-inch square, 8 cups
10 cups boiling water
cinnamon and ginger, optional
½ tsp sea salt
5 Tbsp soy sauce

Red velvet soup – Yield: 8 cups.

1 tsp light sesame oil or olive oil
1 medium onion, thin crescents, 1½ cups
4 medium beets, diced, 3 cups
2 medium carrots, thin quarter rounds, 1½ cups
6 cups boiling water
¼ tsp sea salt
3 Tbsp soy sauce
ground black pepper during cooking, a dash of brown
    rice vinegar at end of cooking, optional

Comments – Puréed vegetable soups are creamy and delicious. Other puréed soup combinations include onion, winter squash, and carrots; or potatoes, celery, and yellow squash.

Sautéed Vegetable Soup with Grain

Procedure – Heat water in a kettle. Heat oil in a pan and sauté onion with a pinch of sea salt until transparent. Add vegetables in the order listed, one kind at a time. Sauté each kind for 1 to 2 minutes. Add boiling water and spices if used. Place grain on top of the vegetables. Sprinkle remaining sea salt on grain. Cover and bring to a boil. Simmer over low heat for the time indicated. Add miso or soy sauce, see page 105.

Cream of celery soup – Simmer 30 minutes. Yield: 9½ cups.

> 1 tsp light sesame oil or olive oil
> 1 large onion, thin crescents, 2 cups
> 4 large celery stalks, thin diagonals, 3 cups
> 8 cups boiling water
> ground black pepper, celery seed, optional
> 1 cup rolled oats
> ¼ tsp sea salt
> 1½ Tbsp miso or 3 Tbsp soy sauce

Russian soup – Wash and drain rice. Roast in a dry skillet (no oil) until browned and popped, 10 to 15 minutes. Simmer soup 1 hour. Yield: 10 cups.

> 1 tsp light sesame oil or olive oil
> 1 medium onion, minced, 1½ cups
> 1 to 2 Tbsp fresh ginger root, finely minced, optional
> 3 medium turnips, diced, 3 cups
> 1 large carrot, thin quarter rounds, 1 cup
> 8 cups boiling water
> 1 cup brown rice, roasted
> ½ tsp sea salt
> 1½ Tbsp miso or 3 Tbsp soy sauce

Comments – Vegetable soup with grain is a variation on the basic sautéed soup. Try other grains such as barley or millet, or soaking the grain for 1 hour instead of roasting before adding to soup. Tofu can be added during the last 5 minutes. Noodles can be added during the last 15 minutes to make a hearty one-pot meal. Try: onion, celery, carrots, millet, and noodles; or onion, garlic, mushrooms, and barley. Soups with whole grains pressure cook well, see page 104.

Sautéed Vegetable Soups with Noodles

Procedure – Heat water in a kettle. Heat oil in a pan and sauté onion with a pinch of sea salt until transparent. Add vegetables in the order listed, one kind at a time. Sauté each kind for 1 to 2 minutes. Add boiling water and spices if used. Sprinkle remaining sea salt on top. Cover and bring to a boil. Simmer 15 minutes. Add noodles and simmer 15 minutes more. Add miso or soy sauce, see page 105.

Cabbage noodle soup – Yield 10 cups.

1 tsp light sesame oil or olive oil
1 medium onion, thin crescents, 1½ cups
2 large celery stalks, thin diagonals, 1½ cups
½ medium cabbage; 5 cups
    core, minced
    leaves, shredded
1 large carrot, matchsticks, 1 cup
8 cups boiling water
ground black pepper, optional
½ tsp sea salt
1 cup whole wheat ribbon noodles
5 tsp miso or 4 Tbsp soy sauce

Summer bean-less minestrone soup – This soup improves the next day. For variation, add 1 cup cooked kidneys beans to this recipe and/or increase the quantity of tomato. Yield: 8 cups.

---

1 tsp light sesame oil or olive oil
1 medium onion, minced, 1½ cups
1 large tomato, diced, 1 cup, see page 79
3 medium zucchini, quarter rounds, 2 cups
2 ears fresh corn, cut off the cob, 2 cups
7 cups boiling water
ground black pepper, crushed garlic, flaked oregano,
     fresh basil, fresh cilantro, optional
½ tsp sea salt
1 cup whole wheat elbow macaroni
4 Tbsp soy sauce

Comments – Noodles can be cooked into almost any kind of soup. Follow the basic procedure and add extra water. Add noodles during the last 15 minutes of simmering. Try these combinations: onion, winter squash, carrots, and whole wheat ribbon noodles garnished with scallions; or onion, celery, buckwheat noodles broken into small pieces, and tofu. Other soups with noodles are listed in the index under noodles.

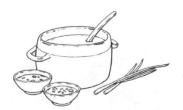

Sautéed Vegetable Soups with Flour

Procedure – Heat water in a kettle. Heat oil in a pan and sauté onion with a pinch of sea salt until transparent or leek greens until bright green. Add vegetables in the order listed, one kind at a time. Sauté each kind for 1 to 2 minutes. Add flour and spices if used, and roast with the vegetables until fragrant, 2 to 3 minutes, stirring constantly. Flour will coat the vegetables. Remove from heat. Add boiling water, using a whisk to smooth lumps. Place over medium heat. Add sea salt. Cover and bring to a boil. Simmer 30 minutes over low heat. Add miso or soy sauce, see page 105.

Creamy leek soup – Wash leeks well before cutting. Yield: 8 cups.

---

2 tsp light sesame oil or olive oil
3 large leeks; 4½ cups
   greens, thin rounds
   whites, thin rounds
1 cup whole wheat flour or brown rice flour
curry powder, ground black pepper, optional
8 cups boiling water
¼ tsp sea salt
1½ Tbsp light miso or 3 Tbsp soy sauce

Creamy cornmeal soup – Yield: 9 cups.

---

2 tsp light sesame oil or olive oil
1 medium onion, thin crescents, 1½ cups
2 medium celery stalks, thin quarter rounds, 1½ cups
2 medium carrots, thin flowers, 1½ cups
1 cup cornmeal or polenta
crushed garlic, cumin powder, dillweed, optional
8 cups boiling water
¼ tsp sea salt
3 Tbsp soy sauce

Comments – Creamy soup with flour is a variation on the basic sautéed soup, roasting flour with sautéed vegetables and then adding boiling water. Other combinations include onion and celery with buckwheat flour; and onion and rutabaga with brown rice flour and garnished with parsley.

Sautéed Vegetable Soups with Arrowroot

Procedure – Heat water in a kettle. Heat oil in a pan and sauté onion with a pinch of sea salt until transparent. Add vegetables in the order listed, one kind at a time. Sauté each kind for 1 to 2 minutes. Add boiling water and spices as desired. Sprinkle remaining sea salt on top. Cover and bring to a boil. Simmer 20 to 25 minutes over low heat. Add dissolved arrowroot powder and stir, simmering until soup is clear and creamy, 1 to 2 minutes. Add soy sauce or miso, see page 105.

Corn and green bean chowder – Yield: 8 cups.

½ tsp light sesame oil or olive oil
1 large onion, minced, 2 cups
4 to 5 large shallots, finely minced, ½ cup, optional
25 large green beans, ½-inch rounds, 2 cups
2 ears of corn, cut off the cob, 2 cups
ground black pepper, optional
6 cups boiling water
¼ tsp sea salt
4 Tbsp arrowroot powder dissolved in ½ cup cold water
1½ Tbsp light miso or 3 Tbsp soy sauce

Comments – Creamy arrowroot soups are variations on the basic sautéed soup, adding dissolved arrowroot after vegetables have cooked tender. Substitute kuzu powder if desired. Other combinations include onion, celery, winter squash and carrots; onion, green peas, and tofu; and leek, celery, and corn.

Miso Soups with Wakame, Boiled

Procedure – Soak wakame in cold water until soft, 10 to 15 minutes. Drain and reserve soaking water. Separate leaves from stems and cut each as directed. In a pot, layer wakame stems and vegetables in the order listed. Add reserved soaking water and cold water, using care not to disturb layers. Cover and bring to a boil. Simmer 20 to 25 minutes over low heat. Add wakame leaves and simmer 5 minutes more. Add miso, see page 105.

Basic miso soup – Yield: 8 cups.

6-inch strip of wakame, soaked in 2 cups water;
    stems, thin rounds
    leaves, ½-inch squares
½ medium cabbage; 4 cups
    core, finely minced
    leaves, shredded
2 medium turnips, diced, 1½ cups
1½ cups reserved soaking water
5 cups water
2 Tbsp barley miso

Cleansing miso soup – Yield: 7 cups.

4-inch strip of wakame, soaked in 2 cups water;
    stems, thin rounds
    leaves, ½-inch squares
1 small daikon radish, thin quarter rounds, 3 cups
1½ cups reserved soaking water
4½ cups water
2 Tbsp barley miso
Garnish: scallions, thin rounds

Comments – Boiling wakame into soup is a variation on the basic boiled vegetable soup. Place softened, chopped wakame stems at the bottom of the pan and layer vegetables from yin at the bottom to yang at the top. Wakame and miso complement each other and produce a hearty nutritious soup. The soup is simmered 20 to 25 minutes in order to cook the wakame stems. The leaves are tender and need only 5 minutes of cooking.

Cornellia Aihara recommended wakame miso soup every day, and to use 2 or 3 kinds of vegetables with 3 parts yin vegetable to 1 part yang vegetable. Try cabbage or bok choy with carrots, daikon, or rutabagas. Try burdock, see page 94, with carrot and onion. Try soaked, sliced shii-take mushrooms, daikon, wakame, garnished with scallions. Miso soup can be made from most of the soup procedures in this chapter.

Miso Soups with Wakame, Sautéed

Procedure – Heat water in a kettle. Soak wakame in cold water until soft, 10 to 15 minutes. Drain and reserve soaking water. Separate leaves from stems and cut each as directed. Heat oil in a pan and sauté onion until transparent. Add vegetables in the order listed, one kind at a time. Sauté each kind until fragrant, 1 to 2 minutes. Place wakame stems on top of the vegetables. Add reserved soaking water and boiling water, using care not to disturb layers. Cover and bring to a boil. Simmer 20 to 25 minutes. Add wakame leaves and simmer another 5 minutes. Add miso, see page 105.

Hearty winter miso soup – Yield: 8 cups

6-inch strip of wakame, soaked in 2 cups water;
  stems, thin rounds
  leaves, ½-inch squares
1 tsp light sesame oil or olive oil
1 large onion, thin crescents, 2 cups
½ small butternut squash, ½-inch squares, 2 cups
2 small turnips, diced, 1 cup
1½ cups reserved soaking water
4 cups boiling water
2 Tbsp barley miso

Spring or summer miso soup – Yield: 8 cups.

6-inch strip of wakame, soaked in 2 cups water;
   stems, thin rounds
   leaves, ½-inch squares
1 tsp light sesame oil or olive oil
1 large onion, thin crescents, 2 cups
1 small bok choy; 3 cups
   whites, thin quarter rounds
   greens, 1-inch squares
1 small carrot, shaved, ½ cup
1½ cups reserved soaking water
5 cups boiling water
2 Tbsp barley miso

Comments – This procedure is a variation on the basic sautéed vegetable soup. Vegetables are sautéed and then boiled with softened, chopped wakame. Try other vegetables for different kinds of miso soup, using one, two, or three kinds of vegetables. Winter squash goes well with daikon radish, beets, or burdock. See kinpira, page 94, for cooking burdock. Summer squash goes well with cabbage, carrots, large green beans, or cabbage hearts. Try a simple soup of only one vegetable like turnips or cabbage. Also, try cooking millet into soup; place ¼ cup washed and drained millet on top of the vegetables before boiling. Increase the water by 2 cups.

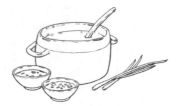

Soups with Fish

Procedure – Heat water in a kettle. Heat oil in a pan and sauté onion with a pinch of sea salt until transparent. Add vegetables in the order listed, one kind at a time. Sauté each kind for 1 to 2 minutes. Add boiling water and any spices used. Sprinkle remaining sea salt on top. Cover and bring to a boil. Simmer 20 minutes over low heat. Add fish and simmer 5 minutes. Mix diluted arrowroot, tahini, miso, and soy sauce, if used; add and stir until clear and creamy.

Potato chowder – See page 79. Yield: 8 cups.

½ tsp light sesame oil
1 large onion, minced, 2 cups
3 medium red potatoes, diced, 4 cups
5 cups boiling water
black pepper, dill weed, garlic, optional
¼ tsp sea salt
½ pound fish fillets, 1-inch pieces, rinsed and dried
2 Tbsp arrowroot diluted in ½ cup rice milk
¼ cup tahini
2 Tbsp light rice miso

Cream of mushroom chowder – Yield: 5 cups.

½ tsp light sesame oil
1 large onion, minced, 2 cups
12 medium mushrooms, sliced, ¼ pound, 2 cups
4 cups boiling water
¼ tsp sea salt
garlic, black pepper, celery seed, optional
½ pound fish fillets, 1-inch pieces, rinsed and dried
2 to 3 Tbsp arrowroot diluted in ¼ cup cold water
2 Tbsp tahini
2 Tbsp soy sauce

Comments – Vegetable soups with fish are a variation on the basic sautéed soup, with fish added during the last 5 minutes of simmering. For variety, cook dumplings or noodles into soup. Also try onion, okra, fresh corn, and fish.

Kombu Soups with Vegetables

Procedure – Place kombu and shiitake mushrooms, if used, in cold water. Cover and bring to a rolling boil. Remove kombu, and mushrooms. Add vegetables and tofu, if used. Bring to a rolling boil again. If using egg, add next, stirring soup constantly while adding. Add soy sauce.

Soba broth with tofu – Yield: 5 cups.

4 cups cold water
4-inch piece kombu
½ pound tofu, ½-inch cubes, 2 cups
4 medium scallions, thin diagonals, 1 cup
4 Tbsp soy sauce

Egg drop soup – See page 154. Yield: 4¼ cups.

4 cups cold water
4-inch piece kombu
2 medium shiitake mushrooms
1 cup minced watercress
1 medium egg, beaten
4 Tbsp soy sauce

Comments – Kombu soup with vegetables is easy to make. It is good served over soba and/or fried fish. Try other combinations such as kombu soup with shredded Chinese cabbage, scallions, and egg. Shiitake mushrooms (more yin) help to balance egg (more yang).

Clear Broths with Kombu

Procedure – Place kombu and shiitake mushrooms, if used, in cold water. Cover and bring to a rolling boil. Remove ingredients immediately and retain for another use. Add soy sauce.

Kombu clear soup (broth for soba) – Yield: 4 cups.

    4-inch piece of kombu
    4 cups cold water
    4 Tbsp soy sauce

Kombu and shiitake mushroom soup – Yield: 4 cups.

    4-inch piece of kombu
    2 medium shiitake mushrooms
    4 cups cold water
    4 Tbsp soy sauce

Comments – Kombu stock is made by bringing water and kombu to a boil and then removing the kombu. It can be used in place of water in any of the soup recipes in this chapter. It can also be used to cook grains. Kombu stock provides a mellow flavor and added nutrients.

Kombu and shiitake mushrooms are used without soaking. When brought to a boil, the flavor is drawn out. Don't boil too long, or stock may become bitter. They can be used to make a second stock. Place in cold water, bring to a boil, and simmer for 15 minutes. Remove. Leftover kombu and shiitake mushrooms can be used in sea vegetable dishes, see page 130. Leftover kombu can be cooked with beans, and leftover shiitake mushrooms can be sliced and cooked into soup.

Serve clear soup with soba or other pasta, garnishing to add flavor or balance. Try thin rounds of scallions or minced parsley; grated carrot or radish; or nori roasted and cut into matchsticks, page 134. For holiday or fancy meals, serve clear soup as a refreshing first course, garnished with a thin quarter slice of lemon, one per bowl.

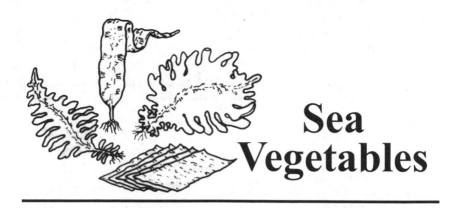

Sea Vegetables

Use – Sea vegetables are high in minerals and add important nutrients to a grain-based diet. Sea vegetables can be used in a variety of ways, from soups to bean dishes to desserts. When used by themselves, sea vegetables are usually served in small amounts as condiments or side dishes.

Rehydrating – Sea vegetables are usually purchased in dried form. Some such as nori and dulse can be used as purchased, while others such as hijiki and arame need to be rehydrated, soaked until softened, before using. Different brands yield different quantities when softened. Some brands are more expensive but yield more when softened than less expensive brands. Hijiki varies considerably.

The recipes included in this chapter call for amounts both in the dry form and in the rehydrated form. If you end up with more or less of the rehydrated sea vegetable than indicated, adjust the quantity of soy sauce. In this case, the indicated quantity of vegetables may be used or adjusted. The proportion of vegetables to sea vegetables is flexible.

Washing – Nori, agar, kombu, and wakame usually don't need washing. Hijiki, arame, and dulse need to be cleaned. Procedures include washing instructions.

Cooking – Thicker sea vegetables (kombu, hijiki, wakame stems) require lengthy cooking to become tender. Thinner and processed sea vegetables (arame, dulse, nori, wakame leaves, agar) cook in shorter times. Soy sauce is used in many sea vegetable dishes to add flavor and balance. Oil is also used for flavor, and is used in sautéing.

125

Hijiki

Procedure – Soak hijiki in water to cover until softened, 10 to 15 minutes. Drain and reserve soaking water. Then wash: Put drained, softened hijiki in a big bowl. Add water to cover. Pour only the hijiki that floats into a sieve without pouring off all the water or hijiki. Add more water and pour off floating hijiki again without pouring off all the water or hijiki. Repeat until all the hijiki has floated and has been poured into the sieve. Sand will have settled to the bottom of the bowl for discarding. Repeat the entire washing process. Drain.

Heat oil in a pan. Add ingredients in the order listed, one kind at a time. Sauté each kind for 1 to 2 minutes. Add reserved soaking water (except for the bottom residue which may contain sand) and extra water to equal the amount called for. Add soy sauce. Cover and leave lid ajar. Bring to a boil. Simmer 20 to 30 minutes over low heat. Remove cover and simmer to reduce remaining liquid.

Hijiki with carrots and sesame seeds – Mix in gomashio at end of cooking. Yield: 4 cups.

2 tsp light sesame oil or olive oil
3 large carrots, thin matchsticks, 3 cups
½ cup hijiki, soaked in 2 cups water; will swell to 2 cups
½ cup reserved soaking water and ½ cup water
2 Tbsp soy sauce
4 Tbsp gomashio, page 186, or roasted sesame seeds, page 185

Hijiki with peanuts – Yield: 2¼ cups.

2 tsp light sesame oil or olive oil
¼ cup raw Spanish peanuts, washed and drained
½ cup hijiki, soaked in 2 cups water; will swell to 2 cups
½ cup reserved soaking water and ½ cup water
2 Tbsp soy sauce

Hijiki with tempeh – Yield: 4 cups.

2 tsp light sesame oil or olive oil
1 large onion, thin crescents, 2 cups
½ cup hijiki, soaked in 2 cups water; will swell to 2 cups
4 ounces tempeh, ½-inch cubes, 1 cup
½ cup reserved soaking water and ½ cup water
3 Tbsp soy sauce

Comments – Hijiki grows in shallow water. All brands contain sand—some more than others. This method of soaking hijiki before washing allows it to soften first so the sand will separate. Then, when washing, some of the water is left in the bowl. The sand will settle to the bottom rather than being poured out with the hijiki. Don't take short cuts when washing hijiki. It may seem faster to rinse the hijiki quickly before rehydrating; however, a quick rinse will not remove the sand.

Arame is similar to hijiki in appearance but has a milder flavor. It grows in 12-inch-long fronds, and is cut into matchsticks before packaging. Hijiki and arame can be substituted for each other. Here are some additional recipe ideas:

Cook with shiitake mushrooms or burdock root. Soak shiitake mushrooms and dice the cap, then simmer with the sea vegetable dish. Shave burdock and cook as on page 94, then proceed as directed above.

Boil tofu for 5 minutes, drain and discard water. Crumble tofu, then mix with the cooked sea vegetable dish. Try onion, carrot, hijiki, shiitake mushroom, and crumbled tofu.

Add cooked noodles. Mix the sea vegetable dish with an equal amount of cooled, cooked noodles and season with more soy sauce.

Arame

Procedure – Soak arame in water until softened, 5 to 10 minutes. Drain and reserve soaking water. Wash arame in the same way as hijiki, one time only, page 126. Heat oil in a pan. Add ingredients in the order listed, one kind at a time. Sauté each kind for 1 to 2 minutes before adding the next one. Add reserved soaking water and soy sauce. Cover and leave lid ajar. Bring to a boil. Simmer 20 to 25 minutes over low heat. Remove cover and simmer to reduce remaining liquid.

Arame with green beans and carrots – Yield: 5 cups.

2 tsp light sesame oil
1 large onion, thin crescents, 2 cups
1 cup arame, soaked in 2 cups water; will swell to 2 cups
25 large green beans, thin diagonals, 2 cups
2 large carrots, thin matchsticks, 2 cups
1 cup reserved soaking water
2 Tbsp soy sauce

Arame with carrots and peanut sauce – Cook arame with all ingredients except peanut butter for 20 minutes. Add diluted peanut butter and cook 5 minutes. Yield: 4 cups.

2 tsp light sesame oil
1 large onion, thin crescents, 2 cups
1 cup arame, soaked in 2 cups water; will swell to 2 cups
2 large carrots, thin matchsticks, 2 cups
1 cup reserved soaking water
2 Tbsp soy sauce
2 Tbsp peanut butter, diluted in 2 Tbsp hot water

Comments – Also try arame with burdock and carrot. For cooking burdock, see page 94. For additional comments, see Hijiki, page 126.

Dulse

Procedure – Gently sort through dulse to remove any shells or rocks. Soak 5 minutes in water. Drain and reserve soaking water. Heat oil in pan. Add ingredients in the order listed, one kind at a time. Saute each kind for 1 to 2 minutes before adding the next one. Add reserved soaking water and soy sauce. Cover and bring to a boil. Simmer 20 to 25 minutes. Remove cover and simmer to reduce remaining liquid.

Dulse with carrots and onions – Yield: 2 cups.

1 tsp light sesame oil or olive oil
1 large onion, thin crescents, 2 cups
1 large carrot, thin matchsticks, 1 cup
¼ cup dulse, soaked in ½ cup water; will swell to ½ cup
½ cup reserved soaking water
2 tsp soy sauce

Dulse with rutabagas – Peel rutabagas if waxed. Yield: 3½ cups.

1 tsp light sesame oil or olive oil
1 large onion, minced, 2 cups
1 pound rutabagas, diced, 3 cups
¼ cup dulse, soaked in ½ cup water; will swell to ½ cup
½ cup reserved soaking water
1 Tbsp soy sauce

Comments – Dulse grows in shallow water. Sometimes there are shells or rocks clinging to the leaves. Clean before soaking as dulse is a delicate sea vegetable and is easier to handle when dry. Dulse and potatoes, see page 79, is a delicious combination and red potatoes may be used in this procedure in place of rutabagas.

Kombu and Nori

Procedure – Soak sea vegetables and shiitake mushrooms, if used, separately in water until softened: sea vegetables, 10 to 15 minutes; shiitake mushrooms, 20 to 25 minutes. Drain kombu and mushrooms, reserve soaking water(s), and slice as directed. Place all ingredients, including reserved soaking water, in a pan. Cover and bring to a boil. Simmer until tender over low heat with lid ajar for time indicated. Remove cover and simmer to reduce remaining liquid.

Kombu with soy sauce – Simmer 30 minutes. Yield: 2 tablespoons.

> 4-inch piece of kombu, soaked in 1 cup water; cut into
>   thin matchsticks after soaking
> 3/4 to 1 tsp soy sauce

Nori with soy sauce – Simmer 15 minutes. Yield: 1½ cups.

> 1 package (10 sheets) nori, torn into 1-inch squares and
>   soaked in 2 cups water
> 4 to 5 tsp soy sauce

Kombu and shiitake mushrooms – Simmer 30 minutes. Yield: ¼ cup.

> 4-inch piece kombu, soaked in 1 cup water; cut into thin
>   matchsticks after soaking
> 2 medium shiitake mushrooms, soaked in 1 cup water;
>   cut after soaking;
>   stems, diced, discard hard uncuttable part
>   caps, thin crescents
> 1½ tsp soy sauce

Kombu and nori – Simmer 30 minutes. Yield: 1½ cups.

4-inch piece kombu, soaked in 1 cup water, cut into thin
    matchsticks after soaking
1 package (10 sheets) nori, torn into 1-inch squares and
    soaked in 2 cups water
5 tsp soy sauce

Comments – Kombu with soy sauce is a chewy and salty condiment. Serve 1 teaspoon at a time on top or along side of rice. Nori with soy sauce is a soft and salty condiment. Serve 2 or more tablespoons per serving. Both will keep 7 to 10 days. Kombu or shiitake mushrooms left over from making soup can be used in these recipes, pages 123-124. There is no need to soak; reduce water by half and cook as above.

Many newer sea vegetable varieties such as sea palm, sea ribbons, and California coast native varieties can be prepared using this procedure: rehydrate, wash, add reserved water and soy sauce, and simmer until done. This basic formula provides a simple sea vegetable condiment.

To make a side dish, saute hearty vegetables such as burdock, carrots, and onions, and then add rehydrated sea vegetables to cook as in the procedures for hijiki or arame, pages 126-128. Add roasted walnuts or almonds to provide texture. Cook with peanuts or tempeh to boost the protein or boil tofu and crumble into the finished dish. Many delicious and original sea vegetable dishes can be made. Have fun!

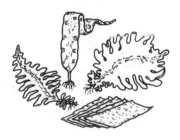

Wakame Salads

Procedure – Soak wakame 10 minutes. Drain. Separate leaves from stems. Chop leaves into ½-inch pieces. Reserve stems and soaking water for soup. Mix dressing. Fold wakame leaves and red onion, if used, in dressing and let stand 5 minutes; then mix with rest of ingredients.

Wakame and cucumber salad – Yield: 2 cups.

1 six-inch piece of wakame, soaked in 1 cup water; will
  swell to 2 Tbsp
Dressing: use procedure on page 166
  1½ tsp light miso
  1 Tbsp almond butter
  2 Tbsp lemon juice
1 medium cucumber, thin half rounds, 2 cups

Wakame, cucumber, and orange salad – Yield: 2½ cups.

1 six-inch piece of wakame, soaked in 1 cup water; will
  swell to 2 Tbsp
Dressing: use procedure on page 166
  1 Tbsp brown rice vinegar
  1 Tbsp soy sauce
  1 tsp toasted sesame oil
2 Tbsp finely minced red onion
2 Tbsp minced celery
1 medium cucumber, thin quarter rounds, 2 cups
1 small tangerine, sectioned and chopped, ¼ cups

Comments – Wakame leaves can be eaten without cooking, but the stems need to be cooked because they are hard. The leaves are soft and are complemented by the crunchy textures of cucumber, celery, and thinly sliced red onion and dressings with soy sauce or light miso, lemon or orange juice, brown rice vinegar, and toasted sesame oil. Wakame salads are best when eaten fresh.

Dulse Salads

Procedure – Gently sort through dulse to remove any shells or rocks. Soak dulse for 5 minutes in liquid to be used in dressing. Then mix in tahini, if used. Mix salad ingredients into dressing in the order listed, one kind at a time.

Dulse salad with carrot, celery, and cucumber – Yield: 3½ cups.

Dressing: ¼ cup dulse
   1 Tbsp lemon juice
   1 Tbsp soy sauce
   1 Tbsp tahini
1 small carrot, grated, ½ cup
2 small celery stalks, diced, 1 cup
1 medium cucumber, thin quarter rounds, 2 cups

Dulse salad with cucumber, celery, and walnut – Yield: 3½ cups.

Dressing: ¼ cup dulse
   2 tsp lemon juice
   2 tsp soy sauce
½ cup roasted walnuts, chopped, pages 183-184
2 small celery stalks, diced, 1 cup
1 medium cucumber, thin quarter rounds, 2 cups

Comments – Dulse is delicate and crumbles when wet, so in these recipes it is mixed into the dressing. Try soaking dulse in any of the mixed salad dressings, page 166, for use in lettuce salads.

Garnishes

Nori, roasted – Roast one side of a sheet of nori by holding it 1 to 2 inches above a low flame or medium-high heat on an electric stove. Pass it back and forth. In 1 to 2 minutes nori will turn green, smell fragrant, and crinkle. Crush, tear into squares, or cut into matchsticks.

Nori, matchsticks – Using scissors, cut one sheet of nori (raw or roasted) in half lengthwise. Cut each half again in half lengthwise. Lay these 4 strips on top of each other. Cut across into very thin matchsticks.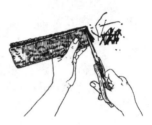

Wakame, roasted – Place dry wakame leaves in dry skillet. Roast over medium to low heat 15 to 20 minutes. Or, place on baking sheet and roast in a 350-degree oven about 10 minutes. Wakame will brown, smell fragrant, and turn crispy. Eat as is or grind to a fine powder in blender or suribachi. Twelve inches of wakame will yield 1 tablespoon of powder. It can be added to gomashio, page 186.

Dulse, roasted – Gently sort through dulse to remove any shells or rocks. Flatten dry dulse and place in a dry skillet. Roast over medium to low heat until dulse is fragrant and crispy, 5 to 7 minutes. Or, place on baking sheet and roast in a 350-degree oven until fragrant, about 5 minutes. Dulse can be eaten raw, but is more flavorful when roasted. Mix roasted dulse with roasted sunflower seeds for a delicious condiment for rice or millet.

Kombu, nori, or dulse, deep-fried – Heat coconut oil (depth of 2 inches) in deep pan. Place individual pieces in oil and fry until crispy and the color changes, 30 seconds to 1 minute. Thicker pieces will take longer. Deep-frying works well for native coast varieties.

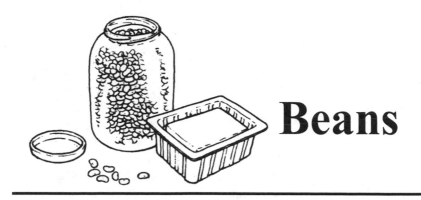

Beans

Use – Beans add flavor, variety, protein, complex carbohydrates, and some fat to a grain-based diet. They can be used in soups, sauces, and side dishes. All whole beans need to be properly cooked for adequate digestion. Here are some tips for whole beans: soak beans; use kombu; pressure cook or boil until completely soft, then cook sea salt into the beans; spice naturally. In preparing bean dishes, there are two steps – cooking until soft by pressure cooking, page 137, or boiling, page 138, and then cooking with sea salt, spices, and vegetables for the completed dish. Fresh beans are covered in Boiled Bean Dishes, page 146.

Cleaning and washing – Sort through beans in small amounts before washing to remove dirt and rocks. To wash: put beans in a pot, add water, swish, and drain. Repeat.

Soaking – Soak dried beans before cooking so the beans will swell. This allows them to cook thoroughly. Soak with kombu in the full quantity of water required for cooking; larger beans require longer soaking times. If preferred, soak without kombu and then discard the soaking water. The soaking water binds some of the gas-forming properties. Add fresh water in the same quantity as the discarded water. Add kombu, soak 15 minutes to hydrate kombu, and then cook. Red lentils, green lentils, and split peas do not require soaking.

Adding kombu – Kombu adds minerals and helps cook beans thoroughly, especially large- and medium-sized beans. After washing beans, add water and kombu, then soak. When cooking, the kombu will become soft and then can be mashed into the beans or removed. Lentils and split peas cook better without kombu.

Adding sea salt – Cook beans until soft before adding sea salt. If sea salt is added early, beans will not become soft. Salt brings out the flavor and adds an alkaline-forming factor. After adding sea salt, cook beans an additional 10 to 30 minutes to dissolve salt. Use ¼ teaspoon sea salt per 1 cup of dried beans.

Cutting and adding vegetables – Cut vegetables into bite-sized pieces, using various cuts of similar size for different vegetables. Cut pieces slightly larger than the bean size to make an attractive dish. Most bean dishes are better if the beans are cooked until soft before adding vegetables. The beans will be cooked thoroughly and the vegetables will be tender but not mushy.

Seasoning – Most bean dishes are cooked with salt. Soy sauce, miso, or other seasonings may be added just before serving to enhance the flavor. If you are cooking a large quantity of beans, season only the portion to be served. The general proportions are 2 to 3 teaspoons soy sauce or 1 to 2 teaspoons miso per 4 cups of any bean dish. Bean dishes cooked with miso need no extra seasoning. Occasionally, herbs and spices such as chili, curry powder, bay leaves, or basil make a nice addition. Avoid those with preservatives or other additives.

Using cooked beans – Cooked beans are versatile. They can adorn pasta or salads or be added to cooked vegetables. Many recipes in this section can be changed by altering the amount of water and serving in a different style. Soups can be made into sauces, or side dishes can be made into soups. See the Leftovers chapter, page 250, for more ideas.

Other beans – Beans and legumes not listed here can be cooked following the simple procedures in this book. Take care with soybeans, however. Dried soybeans are considered one of the hardest beans to cook and digest. Traditional cultures have developed processes to make them more digestible. Products include tofu, tempeh, miso, and soy sauce. Fresh soybeans, known as edamame, have become quite popular in Asian markets and natural food shops. Recipes using tofu and tempeh as well as edamame are included in this chapter.

Pressure-Cooked Beans

Procedure – Sort through beans. Wash and drain. Soak with kombu in the full amount of water. Cover. Place over medium to medium-high heat and bring to full pressure. Slip a heat diffuser under the cooker and turn heat to low. Cook for the time indicated at full pressure.

Large beans – black turtle beans, chickpeas, great northern beans, kidney beans, pinto beans. Soak 6 to 8 hours. Pressure cook 45 minutes. Yield: 5 to 6 cups.

---
2 cups beans
4-inch piece of kombu
4 cups water

Medium beans – black-eyed peas, lima beans, navy beans. Soak 4 to 6 hours. Pressure cook 30 minutes. Yield: 5 cups.

---
2 cups beans
4-inch piece of kombu
4 cups water

Comments – Pressure cooking, as a first step in preparing beans, uses less time and water than boiling. It also deepens the flavor. Soak beans, pressure cook until soft, and then use one of the procedures in this chapter for sautéed or boiled bean dishes as a second step. For more information on using a pressure cooker, see pages 38-41.

Not all beans can be pressure cooked, though. Do not pressure cook lentils, split peas, or soybeans as they may clog the cooker vent. Boil azuki beans for best flavor; they can become bitter if pressure cooked.

Boiled Beans

Procedure – Sort through beans. Wash and drain. Soak, if needed, with kombu, if used, in the full amount of water. Cover and bring to a boil. Simmer for the time indicated over low heat, with lid ajar if necessary to prevent spillover. Add extra water as needed.

Large beans – black turtle beans, chickpeas, great northern beans, kidney beans, pinto beans. Soak 6 to 8 hours. Boil 1½ hours. Yield: 5 to 6 cups.

---

2 cups beans
4-inch piece of kombu
6 cups water

Medium beans – azuki beans, black-eyed peas, lima beans, navy beans. Soak 4 to 6 hours. Boil 50 to 60 minutes. Yield: 5 to 6 cups.

---

2 cups beans
4-inch piece of kombu
6 cups water

Small beans – green lentils, red lentils, split peas. Soaking and kombu are not required for split peas or red lentils. Soaking is optional for green lentils. Boil 20 to 40 minutes. Yield: 5 to 6 cups.

---

2 cups beans
6 cups water

Comments – All beans may be boiled until soft as the first step in preparing bean dishes. Boiling uses more water and takes more time than pressure cooking. After cooking beans until soft, use one of the procedures for sautéed or boiled bean dishes that follow as a second step.

Sautéed Bean Dishes

Procedure – Soak beans with kombu, if used. Cook until soft, page 137 or 138. Heat oil in another pot and sauté onion until transparent. Add vegetables in the order listed, one kind at a time. Sauté each kind for 1 to 2 minutes. Add the additional water. Layer beans and cooking water on top. Sprinkle sea salt on top. Cover and bring to a boil. Simmer 30 minutes over low heat. Add soy sauce.

Navy bean soup – Soak beans with kombu for 4 to 6 hours. Boil 1 hour or pressure cook 30 minutes, then add to vegetables as directed. Yield: 9 cups.

2 cups navy beans, boiled with a 4-inch piece of kombu
    in 6 cups water (4 cups if pressure cooked)
1 tsp light sesame oil or olive oil
1 medium onion, minced, 1½ cups
2 cloves garlic, finely minced, optional
2 medium celery stalks, quarter rounds, 1½ cups
1 medium carrot, thin quarter rounds, ¾ cup
4 or more cups additional water
½ tsp sea salt
2 Tbsp soy sauce, see seasoning, page 136

Azuki beans with onion – Soak azuki beans with kombu for 4 to 6 hours. Boil for 1 hour then follow the basic procedure. Yield: 6½ cups.

2 cups azuki beans, boiled with a 4-inch piece of kombu
    in 6 cups water
½ tsp light sesame oil or olive oil
1 large onion, minced, 2 cups
1 Tbsp fresh ginger, finely minced, optional
¼ tsp salt
½ cup additional water
1 Tbsp soy sauce, see seasoning, page 136

Chickpea spread (hummus) – Soak chickpeas with kombu for 6 to 8 hours. Boil for 1½ hours or pressure cook 45 minutes. After following the basic procedure, purée in a food processor with tahini, lemon juice, and soy sauce until smooth. Yield: 7 cups.

---

2 cups chickpeas, boiled with a 4-inch piece of kombu in
    6 cups water (4 cups if pressure cooked)
1 tsp light sesame oil or olive oil
1 medium onion, minced, 1½ cups
2 or more medium cloves garlic, finely minced
½ cup additional water
½ tsp sea salt
2 Tbsp tahini
4 Tbsp lemon juice
2 Tbsp soy sauce, optional

Lentil soup – Soaking is optional, up to 3 hours. Boil 30 to 40 minutes then add to vegetables as directed. Remove bay leaves when serving. Yield: 10 cups.

---

2 cups lentils, boiled in 6 cups water
1 tsp light sesame oil or olive oil
1 medium onion, minced, 1½ cups
2 Tbsp minced parsley
2 medium celery stalks, quarter rounds, 1½ cups
2 medium carrots, thin quarter rounds, 1½ cups
4 or more cups additional water
2 bay leaves
½ tsp sea salt
2 Tbsp soy sauce, see seasoning, page 136

Comments – These flavorful bean dishes require two pots; one to cook beans until soft, the other to sauté vegetables before adding cooked beans. Vegetables at the bottom help prevent beans from burning. Try black-eyed peas with sautéed onions as a side dish; chickpea, cabbage, carrot, and dumpling soup; kidney bean and roasted cornmeal soup; or azuki bean, onion, tahini, and umeboshi paste as a spread.

Sautéed Bean Dishes with Miso

Procedure – Soak beans with kombu, if used. Cook until soft, page 137 or 138. Heat oil in another pot and sauté onion until transparent. Add vegetables in the order listed, one kind at a time. Sauté each kind for 1 to 2 minutes. Add the additional water. Layer beans and cooking water on top. Place miso on top of beans in lumps. Cover and bring to a boil. Simmer 30 minutes over low heat.

Chili – Soak beans with kombu for 6 to 8 hours. Boil 1½ hours or pressure cook 45 minutes then add to vegetables as directed. Yield: 10 cups.

> 2 cups pinto beans, boiled with a 4-inch piece of kombu
>   in 6 cups water (4 cups if pressure cooked)
> 1 tsp light sesame oil or olive oil
> 1 large onion, minced, 2 cups
> 2 large tomatoes, diced, 2 cups, see page 79
> 1 medium green pepper, diced, ¾ cup
> chili powder, cumin, crushed garlic, optional
> 4 cups additional water
> 4 Tbsp soybean or dark barley miso

Kidney beans with miso – Soak kidney beans with kombu for 6 to 8 hours. Boil 1½ hours or pressure cook 45 minutes, then follow basic procedure. Yield: 5 cups.

> 2 cups kidney beans, boiled with a 4-inch piece of
>   kombu in 6 cups water (4 cups if pressure cooked)
> 1 tsp light sesame oil or olive oil
> 1 large onion, minced, 2 cups
> ½ cup additional water
> 2 to 3 Tbsp soybean or dark barley miso

Comments – This variation on the basic sautéed bean dish procedure uses miso cooked into the beans, making the dish rich and dark.

Sautéed Bean Dishes with Spices

Procedure – Soak beans with kombu, if used. Cook until soft, page 137 or 138. Heat oil in another pot and sauté onion until transparent. Add vegetables in the order listed, one kind at a time. Sauté each kind for 1 to 2 minutes. Add spices. Sauté briefly to enhance flavor. Add the additional water. Layer beans and bean cooking water on top. Sprinkle sea salt on top of the beans. Cover and bring to a boil. Simmer 30 minutes over low heat. Add soy sauce if used.

Split pea curry sauce – Boil peas for 1 hour then add to vegetables as directed. Yield: 6½ cups.

---

2 cups split peas, boiled in 6 cups water
1 tsp light sesame oil or olive oil
1 large onion, minced, 2 cups
1 large celery stalk, thin quarter rounds, ¾ cup
½ tsp curry powder, or more
1 cup additional water
½ tsp sea salt
2 Tbsp soy sauce, optional, see seasoning, page 136

Red lentil dal – Boil red lentils for 20 minutes then add to vegetables as directed. Yield: 7 to 9 cups.

---

2 cups red lentils, boiled in 6 cups water
1 tsp light sesame oil or olive oil
1 large onion, minced, 2 cups
2 medium garlic cloves, finely minced, or more
1 large celery stalk, thin quarter rounds, ¾ cup
2 medium red potatoes, diced, 2½ cups, optional, see page 79
1 large carrot, quarter rounds, 1 cup
½ tsp cumin, or more
¼ tsp coriander, or more
½ cup additional water
½ tsp sea salt

Mexican beans – Soak beans with kombu for 6 to 8 hours. Boil for 1½ hours or pressure cook for 45 minutes then follow basic procedure. Yield: 6 cups.

2 cups pinto beans, boiled with a 4-inch piece of kombu
  in 6 cups water (4 cups if pressure cooked)
1 tsp light sesame oil or olive oil
1 medium onion, minced, 1½ cups
2 medium garlic cloves, finely minced, or more
½ tsp chili powder, or more
½ cup additional water
½ tsp sea salt

Black turtle bean soup – Soak black turtle beans with kombu for 6 to 8 hours. Boil for 1½ hours or pressure cook for 45 minutes then add to vegetables as directed. Yield: 10 cups.

2 cups black turtle beans boiled with a 4-inch piece of
  kombu in 6 cups water (4 if pressure cooked)
1 tsp light sesame oil or olive oil
1 large onion, minced, 2 cups
2 to 3 cloves garlic, finely minced, or more
1 stalk celery, thin quarter rounds, 1 cup
1 large carrot, thin quarter rounds, 1 cup
½ tsp cumin, or more
¼ tsp coriander, or more
2 Tbsp fresh parsley, minced
2 Tbsp fresh cilantro, minced
4 cups additional water
½ tsp sea salt

Comments – This procedure is a variation on the basic sautéed bean dish. Spices or herbs are added and sautéed briefly to increase flavor. Garlic enhances almost all bean dishes. For another recipe, try chickpeas with garlic, fresh basil, parsley, and cilantro.

Baked Beans

Procedure – Soak beans with kombu, if used. Cook until soft, page 137 or 138. Heat oil and sauté onion until transparent. Add any other vegetables, one kind at a time, and sauté for 1 to 2 minutes. Add beans and bring to a boil. Mix miso with mustard, tomato, and barley malt, if used, and add to beans. Cover. Place in oven and bake at 350 degrees for 1 hour.

> **Boston baked beans** – Soak beans with kombu for 6 to 8 hours. Boil 1½ hours or pressure cook 45 minutes then add to vegetables as directed. Yield: 5½ cups.

---

2 cups great northern beans, boiled with a 4-inch piece
    of kombu in 6 cups water (4 cups if pressure cooked)
1 tsp light sesame oil or olive oil
1 large onion, minced, 2 cups
3 to 4 Tbsp soybean or dark barley miso
2 Tbsp wet mustard
½ cup tomato sauce, optional, see page 79
2 Tbsp barley malt, optional

Comments – This procedure is a variation on the basic sautéed bean dish procedure. Baked beans are rich and warming. Sauté vegetables in ovenware for ease in preparation, or sauté vegetables, mix with beans and other ingredients, and bake in a casserole pan. Vary this recipe and include other vegetables such as celery, garlic, mushrooms, or carrots.

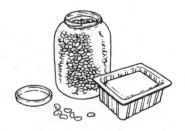

Boiled Bean Dishes

Procedure – Soak beans with kombu, if used. Cook until soft, page 137 or 138. Using the same pot, add the additional water. Mix with beans so water is at the bottom of the pot. Add vegetables. Sprinkle sea salt on top. Cover and bring to a boil. Simmer 30 minutes over low heat, using a heat diffuser if needed. Add soy sauce if used.

Simple beans – Simmer with sea salt for 15 to 20 minutes. Serve as is or add to cooked pasta dishes or salads. Yield: 5 to 6 cups.

2 cups black-eyed peas, chickpeas, or kidney beans, boiled with a 4-inch piece of kombu in 6 cups water (4 cups if pressure cooked)
½ cup additional water
½ tsp sea salt

Minestrone – Soak navy or lima beans with kombu for 4 to 6 hours. Boil for 1 hour or pressure cook for 30 minutes then follow basic procedure. Simmer soup 15 minutes, add noodles and simmer 15 minutes more. Yield: 9 cups.

½ cup navy or lima beans, boiled with a 1-inch piece of kombu in 2 cups water (1½ cups if pressure cooked)
6 or more cups additional water
1 medium onion, minced, 1½ cups
1 medium celery stalk, quarter rounds, ¾ cup
½ small cabbage, squares, 2½ cups
1 medium ear of corn, cut off the cob, 1 cup
1 large carrot, quarter rounds, 1 cup
garlic, black pepper, dill weed, bay leaf, optional
½ to ¾ tsp sea salt
1 cup whole wheat elbow macaroni
3 Tbsp soy sauce, see seasoning, page 136

Split pea soup – Boil split peas for 1 hour, then add vegetables as directed. Yield: 10 cups.

---

2 cups split peas, boiled in 6 cups water
4 or more cups additional water
1 large onion, minced, 2 cups
2 medium celery stalks, quarter rounds, 1½ cups
2 medium carrots, thin quarter rounds, 1½ cups
½ tsp sea salt
5 tsp soy sauce, see seasoning, page 136

Azuki beans with winter squash – Soak azuki beans with kombu for 4 to 6 hours. Boil 45 minutes, then add vegetables as directed. Yield: 9 cups.

---

2 cups azuki beans, cooked with a 4-inch piece of
    kombu in 6 cups water
½ cup additional water
1 large butternut squash, 1-inch squares, 8 cups
½ tsp sea salt

Fresh beans and peas: black-eyed peas, fava beans, green soybeans (edamame), green peas, lima beans – If beans are in the pod, they can be shelled. Green soybeans are often cooked in the pod and shelled after cooking. There is no need to use kombu. Boil beans until tender, from 5 to 30 minutes, until softened. Add additional water as needed. Add sea salt and cook another 10 minutes. Yield: 2 cups.

---

2 cups fresh beans
water to cover
¼ tsp sea salt

Comments – Cook the beans until soft, and then continue to cook in the same pan, making the dish as simple or fancy as desired. If using a pressure cooker, do not lock the cover on the cooker while boiling; use a different lid. Also try simple beans cooked with onion.

Boiled Bean Dishes with Tahini

Procedure – Soak beans with kombu, if used. Cook until soft, page 137 or 138. Using the same pot, add the additional water. Mix with beans so water is at the bottom of the pot. Add vegetables. Sprinkle sea salt on top. Cover and bring to a boil. Simmer 30 minutes over low heat with heat diffuser if necessary. Dilute tahini and soy sauce in ½ cup of the hot broth, then add and remove from heat.

Chickpea sauce – Soak chickpeas with kombu for 6 to 8 hours. Boil 1½ hours or pressure cook 45 minutes, then follow basic procedure. Yield: 10 cups.

---

2 cups chickpeas, boiled with a 4-inch piece of kombu in
    6 cups water (4 cups if pressure cooked)
1 cup additional water
1 large celery stalk, thin quarter rounds, 1 cup
1 small cabbage, shredded, 5 cups
1 large onion, minced, 2 cups
1 large carrot, quarter rounds, 1 cup
½ tsp sea salt
3 Tbsp tahini
3 Tbsp soy sauce

Lentil spread – Soaking is optional, up to 3 hours. Boil 40 minutes, then follow basic procedure. After cooking, mash or purée spread in a food processor. Yield: 6 cups.

---

2 cups lentils, boiled in 6 cups water
½ cup additional water
1 medium onion, diced, 1½ cups
2 medium celery stalks, thin quarter rounds, 1½ cups
½ tsp sea salt
garlic, curry powder, thyme leaf, optional
2 Tbsp tahini
2 Tbsp soy sauce

Comments – This procedure is a variation on the basic boiled bean dish procedure. Diluted tahini makes these dishes creamy. Also try lima beans with onion, celery, and tahini.

Scrambled Tofu

Procedure – Slice tofu into ¼-inch-thick rectangular pieces. Remove excess water by pressing between two flat surfaces, such as two cutting boards. Paper toweling under the tofu will speed the process. Weight with a heavy pan or a bottle of water for 5 minutes. Remove tofu and mash. Heat oil. Add onion and sea salt. Sauté until transparent. Add other vegetables in the order listed. Sauté each kind briefly, 1 to 2 minutes. Add tofu and millet, if used. Sauté 1 to 2 minutes. Cover. Steam 5 minutes over low heat. Add soy sauce.

Scrambled tofu with vegetables – Yield: 3 cups.

½ pound tofu, 2 cups
2 tsp light sesame oil or olive oil
1 small onion, minced, 1 cup
⅛ tsp sea salt
1 cup fresh green peas or finely chopped green beans
1 small carrot, finely minced, ½ cup
1 Tbsp soy sauce

Scrambled tofu with millet – Yield: 3 cups.

½ pound tofu, 2 cups
2 tsp light sesame oil or olive oil
1 small onion, finely minced, 1 cup
⅛ tsp sea salt
2 small celery stalks, finely minced, 1 cup
½ cup cooked millet
1 Tbsp soy sauce

Comments – This procedure uses tofu in combination with vegetables and cooked grains or pastas to make a quick dish or one-pot meal. Many possible dishes can be made such as: cooked buckwheat, tofu, and scallion; or finely minced ginger, cooked rice, onion, tofu, and soy sauce. Herbs and spices complement tofu well and can be used liberally; ginger and garlic are delicious. Curry powder or turmeric adds a yellowish color reminiscent of scrambled eggs. The above recipes are mild in seasoning, so add more flavoring as desired.

Tofu Burgers

Procedure – Slice tofu into ¼-inch-thick rectangular pieces. Remove excess water by pressing between two flat surfaces, such as two cutting boards. Paper toweling under the tofu will speed the process. Weight with a heavy pan or a bottle of water for 5 minutes. Remove tofu and mash. Mix with other ingredients. (A food processor can be used to mince vegetables.) Mixture should hold its shape without being too wet or too dry. Form into patties, 3 to 4 inches in diameter, ½-inch thick. Heat oil in a skillet. Pan-fry 4 to 5 burgers at a time. Cover skillet for the first side, and fry for 7 minutes. Uncover for the second side, and fry for 5 minutes. Add more oil to skillet for second and third batches.

Tofu burgers – Serve with Soy and ginger sauce, page 176. Yield: 10 burgers.

½ pound firm or extra firm tofu, 2 cups
½ small onion, finely minced, ½ cup
1 small celery stalk, finely minced, ½ cup
½ small carrot, grated, ¼ cup
¼ tsp sea salt
½ to ¾ cup whole wheat or whole wheat pastry flour
1 Tbsp coconut oil for skillet

Tofu millet burgers – Serve with Soy and ginger sauce, page 176. Yield: 14 burgers.

½ pound firm or extra firm tofu, 2 cups
1 cup cooked millet, mashed
1 small onion, finely minced, 1 cup
1 small celery stalk, finely minced, ½ cup
¼ tsp sea salt
½ cup whole wheat or whole wheat pastry flour
1 Tbsp coconut for skillet

Comments – Tofu burgers are delicious served with pasta or made into sandwiches with whole wheat bread or buns and lettuce or pressed cabbage. For variation make Tofu burgers with cooked rice or cooked buckwheat, or add minced carrot, parsley, red onion, or other vegetables. For more seasoning, add miso to the mixture or herbs such as oregano, garlic, or curry powder. See pages 16-17 on use of oil.

Pan-Fried or Baked Tofu

Procedure – Slice tofu into ¼- to ½-inch-thick rectangular pieces. Remove excess water by pressing between two flat surfaces, such as two cutting boards. Paper toweling under the tofu will speed the process. Weight with a heavy pan or a bottle of water for 5 minutes. Remove.

To marinate: place tofu in marinade for 3 to 4 hours, turning occasionally until the marinade is absorbed.

To fry: prepare coating. Dip each piece in coating. Heat oil in skillet. Pan-fry tofu until golden, 3 to 4 minutes on each side.

To bake: prepare marinade ingredients. Place tofu and marinade on oiled baking sheet. Bake at 350 degrees for 15 to 20 minutes until marinade is absorbed; flip after 10 minutes.

Simple and quick pan-fried tofu – Yield: 6 pieces.

½ pound tofu
½ cup arrowroot powder, buckwheat flour, or whole
    wheat pastry flour for coating
1 to 2 Tbsp coconut oil for frying

Marinated pan-fried or baked tofu – Yield: 12 pieces.

1 pound tofu
Marinade: 3 Tbsp soy sauce
    1 Tbsp freshly squeezed ginger juice
    1 Tbsp toasted sesame oil
Coating: 4 Tbsp gomashio
    4 Tbsp arrowroot powder
2 to 3 Tbsp coconut oil for frying

Comments – In this procedure, tofu is pressed to remove excess water. Tofu will absorb more flavor in the marinade and there will be less moisture to cause the oil to spatter when frying. Simple and quick pan-fried tofu is fast to prepare. Serve with soy sauce on top, with Scallion miso, page 91, or Soy and ginger sauce, page 176. Or, sliver after frying and serve on buckwheat noodles.

Marinated pan-fried tofu is more flavorful but takes longer to prepare as it needs time to marinate. This step can be done overnight in the refrigerator. To vary the marinade, add other flavorings or liquids such as granulated garlic, onion, black pepper, or brown rice vinegar.

Baked tofu is drier than pan-fried tofu. Both are delicious in sandwiches. See pages 16-17 on use of oil.

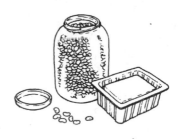

Pan-Fried or Deep-Fried Tempeh

Procedure – Slice tempeh into thin rectangles and marinate for 5 to 10 minutes or longer. Drain excess liquid and reserve.

To pan-fry: Heat oil in a skillet. Pan-fry until golden, 2 to 3 minutes for each side. Add reserved marinade and additional water so there is ½-inch of liquid in the pan. Cover pan. Simmer 10 to 15 minutes until liquid is gone.

To deep-fry: Use a ½-quart stainless steel pan and add coconut oil to a depth of 2 inches. Heat. Add 1 piece of tempeh to test the temperature of the oil. It should rise to the surface and fry. Add 5 or more pieces so tempeh can cook freely without crowding. Cook each side for 2 to 3 minutes. Remove with tongs to a strainer or toweling.

Pan-fried or deep-fried tempeh – Yield: 8 pieces.

---

8 ounces of tempeh
Marinade: 2 Tbsp soy sauce
    2 Tbsp water or lemon juice or 1 to 2 tsp ginger juice
        (grate fresh ginger root on a Japanese grater,
        squeeze out juice, discard pulp)
coconut oil for frying

Comments – Tempeh is delicious when fried in oil. Marinate it first to add more flavor. Vary the marinade by adding granulated garlic or cumin. Serve with pressed cabbage or sauerkraut or in a sandwich. Coconut oil complements tempeh for frying. It remains stable at high temperatures and is well suited for deep frying. See pages 16-17 on the use of oil.

Sautéed Tempeh with Vegetables

Procedure – Cube or crumble tempeh. Marinate 5 to 10 minutes. Drain excess liquid and reserve. Heat oil in pan. Sauté onion until transparent. Add vegetables in the order listed. Sauté each kind briefly, 1 to 2 minutes. Add tempeh and sauté for 1 to 2 minutes. Add reserved marinade and additional water so there is ½-inch of liquid in the pan. Cover. Simmer 10 to 15 minutes, then remove cover and simmer to reduce remaining liquid.

Tempeh with mushrooms – Yield: 1½ cups.

4 ounces of tempeh
Marinade: 2 Tbsp soy sauce and 2 Tbsp water
2 tsp light sesame oil, olive oil, or coconut oil
1 small onion, minced, 1 cup
12 medium mushrooms, thin lengthwise slices, ¼ pound,
   2 cups
water

Tempeh with red pepper – Yield: 2½ cups.

8 ounces of tempeh
Marinade: 3 Tbsp soy sauce and 2 Tbsp water
2 tsp light sesame oil, olive oil, or coconut oil
1 small onion, minced, 1 cup
1 large red bell pepper, diced, 1 cup
water

Comments – Tempeh sautéed with vegetables makes a flavorful side dish or topping for pasta or salad. For variations, cook tempeh with onion, onion and garlic, or Burdock and carrots, see page 94. Tempeh is also delicious with arame or hijiki. See Sea Vegetables chapter.

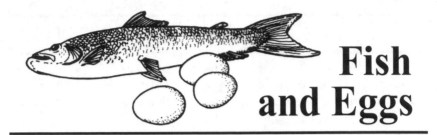

Fish and Eggs

Use – Although optimum health may be obtained without the use of animal foods and a majority of macrobiotic practitioners are vegetarian, many include small amounts of fish and some include eggs occasionally. Both are included in this chapter to provide practical information on how to prepare them in a balanced way.

Fish – Buy fish as fresh as possible and rinse before cooking to freshen. Pat dry with a paper towel. If fish is frozen, thaw in the refrigerator, then rinse and pat dry. Many recipes in this chapter use ginger juice and soy sauce to marinate fish. Both ginger juice and soy sauce add flavor as well as an alkaline-balancing factor. Fish is considered yang, so using ginger or lemon juice, and serving with lemon slices, grated daikon radish, or salad adds a yin quality. To make ginger juice: Grate fresh ginger with a Japanese or other fine grater. Squeeze out the juice and discard the pulp.

Fish cooks quickly; it is done when the flesh becomes opaque and begins to flake. Fillets cook faster than whole fish, and thinner pieces cook faster than thicker ones.

Eggs – Eggs are high in sodium and fat and are considered more yang. Used on occasion, they provide extra nutrients for oneself, growing kids, expecting and nursing mothers, and guests. Choose fertile eggs from free-ranging chickens. Use eggs in baked goods, side dishes, and even soups. Balance egg dishes by cooking or serving with more yin items such as sprouts, peppers, or fruit, especially citrus.

Pan-Fried Fish

Procedure – Rinse and dry fish and cut into serving-sized pieces. Pour marinade over fish. Let stand 5 minutes. Turn fish over and let stand another 5 minutes. Remove from marinade. Cover with coating. Heat oil in a skillet. Fry fish 2 to 3 minutes, with cover on pan. Turn and fry the second side without cover for 2 to 3 minutes or until browned.

Pan-fried perch

1 pound perch fillets or other fresh fish
Marinade: 2 Tbsp soy sauce and 2 Tbsp freshly squeezed
    lemon juice or freshly grated ginger juice, page 154
Coating: arrowroot flour, fine cornmeal, or whole wheat
    pastry flour
1 Tbsp coconut oil for skillet

Comments – Use fillets for pan-frying. Fresh tuna, red snapper, and tilapia are delicious. Other seasonings can be added to the marinade such as granulated garlic or onion, or liquids such as brown rice vinegar. Seasonings such as gomashio, cumin, curry powder, garlic powder, or black pepper can be added to the coating.

Whole fish can be pan-fried, too. Cut down the backbone and open to marinate. Allow more time for frying. Fish is done when the flesh begins to flake.

Serve fried fish with lemon slices and/or salad; or with soba in Kombu and shiitake mushroom soup, page 124.

Broiled Fish

Procedure – Rinse and dry fish. For fillets, cut into serving-sized pieces. For whole fish, slit down backbone and open. Pour marinade over fish. Let stand 5 minutes. Turn fish over and let stand another 5 minutes. Remove from marinade and place on oiled broiling pan. Place under broiler and watch carefully. Thicker fish should be turned once. Brush extra marinade on the fish when turning. Remove when flesh begins to flake.

> **Broiled salmon or halibut** – Broil 4 to 5 minutes each side.
>
> ---
>
> 1 pound salmon or halibut
> Marinade: 2 Tbsp soy sauce and 2 Tbsp freshly squeezed
> lemon juice or freshly grated ginger juice, page 154
>
> ---

Comments – Broiling uses heat as high as 500 to 600 degrees. Food is placed under the heat so it is cooked from above. The closer the fish is to the heat, the faster it will cook. Thin fillets can broil in 3 to 4 minutes if close to the heat, but may require up to 8 minutes if further from the heat. Since the size and kind of fish and ovens vary, watch carefully so as not to overcook fish. Remove immediately when the flesh begins to flake.

Salmon is high in fat and is enhanced with broiling. Fish with less fat such as halibut broil well too. If desired, drizzle with olive oil when removing from heat for flavor and to help retain moisture.

Also, if desired, salt and pepper and herbs such as basil, dill, or sage can be sprinkled on fish before broiling.

Baked Fish

Procedure – Rinse and dry fish. Pour marinade over fish. Let stand 5 minutes. Turn fish over and let stand another 5 minutes. Place fish and marinade in baking dish. Bake at 350 degrees until flesh begins to flake.

Baked trout – Bake 30 minutes.

2 trout, whole
Marinade (use 2 Tbsp marinade per 8 ounces of fish):
    1 Tbsp soy sauce and 1 Tbsp freshly squeezed lemon
        juice or freshly grated ginger juice, page 154

Baked orange roughy – Bake 15 to 20 minutes.

1 pound orange roughy fillets, ½-inch thick
Marinade: ¼ tsp sea salt or ½ tsp soy sauce
    2 tsp freshly grated ginger juice, page 154
    dill weed, granulated onion, and granulated garlic,
        optional
1 Tbsp olive oil, drizzle on fish when serving

Comments – Any fish can be baked with good results. Whole fish and thicker pieces of fish need to bake longer. Thin fillets such as orange roughy can bake in 15 minutes, while thick fillets such as salmon or halibut may take 30 minutes. Whole fish such as trout may require 30 minutes, while a whole salmon could take up to 1 hour. Baking is a preferred way to prepare whole fish as the heat gently surrounds the fish, and the skin helps keep the fish tender and moist. If desired, cover the baking dish for additional retention of heat and moisture.

Baked Fish with Vegetables

Procedure – Rinse and dry fish. Pour marinade over fish and let stand 5 minutes. Turn fish over and let stand another 5 minutes. Sauté vegetables in oil for 4 to 5 minutes. Place fish, marinade, and vegetables in oiled casserole dish. Add boiling water if needed so ¼ inch of liquid is at bottom. Cover dish. Bake 25 to 30 minutes at 350 degrees, until flesh begins to flake.

Baked fish with onion

> ½ pound trout or other fish
> Marinade: 1 Tbsp soy sauce and 1 Tbsp freshly squeezed
>   lemon juice or freshly grated ginger juice, page 154
> 1 tsp coconut oil
> 1 large onion, minced, 2 cups
> boiling water as needed

Baked fish with carrots and potatoes – Sauté vegetables by adding in the order listed.

> 1 pound salmon fillet, or other fish
> Marinade: 2 Tbsp soy sauce and 2 Tbsp freshly squeezed
>   lemon juice or freshly grated ginger juice, page 154
> 1 tsp coconut oil
> 1 large onion, minced, 2 cups
> 3 medium potatoes, diced, 4 cups, see page 79
> 2 small carrots, shaved, 1 cup
> boiling water as needed

Comments – Bake fish (fillets or whole) with vegetables for a hearty and balanced dish. Cover dish for moisture and heat retention. Try also yellow squash, green peppers, or fresh mushrooms.

Steamed Fish

Procedure – Rinse and dry fish. Add water to the pan to a depth of ¼ inch. Bring to a boil. Add sea salt. Add fish and sprinkle basil on top. Cover. Steam fish 3 to 4 minutes until flesh begins to flake.

Steamed cod

1 pound cod fillets or other whole fresh fish, or fish fillets
water as needed
pinch of sea salt
½ tsp basil

Comments – Steaming works best for freshly caught or one-day-old fish. For "older" fish, soak in salt water to freshen as follows: Dissolve 1 tablespoon sea salt in 1 cup of water. Add fish, soak for 30 minutes, rinse and dry.

Fillets steam well for a light summertime dish. They steam quickly; don't overcook, as fish can become tough. Try adding 1 tablespoon lemon juice to the boiling water or steaming fish with parsley. When serving, dress with a sauce or dressing that contains oil such as Olive oil and umeboshi vinegar dressing, page 167.

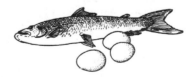

Scrambled Eggs

Procedure – Lightly beat eggs. Add other ingredients. Mix well. Heat oil in a skillet. Add mixture. Fry over medium heat, stirring constantly until the eggs are cooked through and are a dull yellow, 3 to 4 minutes. For mixtures with tofu and millet, cover pan and steam an additional 2 to 3 minutes.

Scrambled eggs – Yield: ½ cup.

2 eggs
1 Tbsp lemon or 2 Tbsp orange juice, freshly squeezed
pinch sea salt or ¼ tsp soy sauce
2 tsp light sesame oil or olive oil for skillet

Scrambled egg with tofu – Yield: 2 cups.

1 egg
½ pound tofu, pressed and mashed, page 149, 2 cups
1 tsp lemon or 1 Tbsp orange juice, freshly squeezed
curry powder, garlic, optional
2 tsp soy sauce
2 tsp light sesame oil or olive oil for skillet

Scrambled egg with millet – Yield: 1¼ cups.

1 egg
1 cup cooked and cooled millet, mashed
4 medium scallions, thin rounds, 1 cup
1 tsp lemon or 1 Tbsp orange juice, freshly squeezed
½ tsp soy sauce
2 tsp light sesame oil or olive oil for skillet

Comments – Balance and enhance eggs with citrus juice and soy sauce. Variation: use cooked rice and add chopped bean sprouts.

Scrambled Eggs with Vegetables

Procedure – Heat oil in a skillet. Sauté onion until transparent. Add vegetables. Sauté for 1 to 2 minutes. Add water, tofu and/or grain if used, and sea salt. Cover. Steam 5 to 7 minutes until water is gone. Add egg. Scramble until egg is cooked, 3 to 4 minutes.

Scrambled egg with red pepper and tofu. Yield: 3½ cups.

2 tsp light sesame oil or olive oil
1 large onion, minced, 2 cups
1 large red bell pepper, diced, 1 cup
¼ cup water
½ pound tofu, pressed and mashed, page 149, 2 cups
pinch of sea salt
1 egg, beaten

Scrambled egg with rice and celery. Yield: 3 cups.

2 tsp light sesame oil or olive oil
1 large onion, minced, 2 cups
1 large celery stalk, diced, 1 cup
¼ cup water
1 cup cooked brown rice or wild rice
pinch of sea salt
1 egg, beaten

Comments – Use egg in combination with vegetables, cooked grains, and tofu to make delicious one-pot meals or side dishes. Use finely cut vegetables for best results. Other combinations: onion and egg; broccoli, onion, and egg; tofu, cooked buckwheat, sweet potatoes, eggs, scallions.

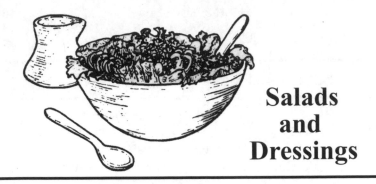

Salads
and
Dressings

Vegetables – Salads provide lightness to a meal and are especially appropriate in hot climates (yang) or when serving yang foods such as fish because raw salads are generally more yin. Use young fresh vegetables for tender and crisp salads. Wash vegetables well and dry completely. Pat dry with a towel if necessary or use a salad spinner.

Dressings – Salad dressings add flavor and nutrition to salads. They can be thick or thin depending on use or preference. Generally, thinner dressings are mixed with raw or medley salads, or served separately. Thicker dressings are mixed with vegetables or used as dips. Make dressings in small amounts for one meal. If boiled, sautéed, or heated, let dressing cool before mixing or serving with salad. Generally, use 1 tablespoon of dressing per 1 cup of salad.

Sea Salt – Traditionally, macrobiotics considered it preferable to cook sea salt into food rather than to shake it on "raw" while eating. (For more information on sea salt, see page 261.) In this chapter, there is some variation from this idea. Raw sea salt is used in some dressings and condiments. In these recipes, oil coats the sea salt, making it easier to digest.

Other salads – The recipes in this section are only a sample of the many salads you can make. Use other vegetable combinations and dressings to create your own salads. Other salad recipes can be found in the Pickles and Pressed Salads chapter, pages 188-199, and Sea Vegetables chapter, pages 125-134.

Raw Salads, Tossed

Procedure – Gently combine washed and dried salad ingredients. For lettuce salad, use up to ¾ of the total ingredients as lettuce(s). Cut vegetables very thin so that when tossing, the salad will be uniform rather than having big pieces fall to the bottom of the salad bowl. Mix dressing of choice, toss with salad, or serve separately, see pages 166-170.

Tossed salad – Combine 3 or 4 ingredients.

lettuce, torn into bite-sized squares
bitter greens such as arugula, torn into bite-sized pieces
young baby greens from bok choy, chard, or others, torn
    into bite-sized pieces
cabbage, red or green, shredded
cucumber, thin rounds, half-rounds, or quarter-rounds
radish, thin rounds or half-rounds
small celery stalks, thin quarter rounds
carrot, grated, thin rounds, or matchsticks
scallion, thin rounds
sprouts, any kind, whole
red bell pepper, diced or thin crescents
young zucchini or yellow squash, thin rounds or half-
    rounds
young fresh beets, turnips, kohlrabi, or daikon radish,
    grated
red onion, thin crescents
jicama, thin matchsticks
avocado, chunks
tomato, chunks, optional, see page 79

Comments – Raw salad is easy to prepare for a hot summer day or as part of an elaborate meal. There are many vegetables that can be used. Some such as beets, turnips, and summer squash can be used raw if young and fresh. Others such as kohlrabi are more appealing raw than cooked. Still others such as snow peas can be lightly boiled, page 100.
    Another way to assemble a salad is to toss most of the ingredients

and then lay heavier items such as avocado and tomato on top. Add items such as cooked chickpeas, page 145, or Marinated baked tofu, page 151, for extra nutrition.

Raw Salads, Layered

Procedure – Layer ingredients in the order listed. Mix dressing of choice and serve separately.

Lettuce, cucumber, and sunflower salad – Yield: 6 cups.

½ medium lettuce, torn into bite-sized squares, 4 cups
½ small carrot, grated, ¼ cup
1 medium cucumber, half-rounds, 2 cups
¼ cup roasted sunflower seeds, pages 183-184
Dressing: Soy sauce dressing (use lemon juice), page 166

Lettuce, radish, and avocado salad – Yield: 5 cups.

½ medium lettuce, torn into bite-sized squares, 4 cups
4 large radishes, thin rounds, ½ cup
2 medium scallions, thin rounds, ½ cup
1 avocado, chunks, ¾ cup
Dressing: Umeboshi paste dressing (use lime juice and
    tahini), page 166

Comments – Layering is practical when serving 1 or 2 people, or when using ingredients such as avocado or seeds that would mash or fall to the bottom of the bowl when tossing. Layer salads in individual bowls and use different colors for appeal. Serve with a simple, pourable dressing.

Raw Salads, Tossed with Dressing

Procedure – Make dressing. Cool for 5 minutes. Gently mix salad ingredients into the dressing in the order listed, one kind at a time. Let stand 10 minutes before serving to allow flavors to mingle.

Lettuce, carrot, and sprouts salad – Yield: 6 cups.

Dressing: Onion and soy sauce dressing (use brown rice
vinegar), 1½ cups, page 168
1 cup alfalfa sprouts
1 small carrot, grated, ½ cup
1 small lettuce, torn into bite-sized squares, 4 cups

Cucumber and avocado salad – Yield: 2½ cups.

Dressing: Avocado dressing, ¾ cup, page 167
1 medium scallion, thin rounds, ¼ cup
1 small celery stalk, thin quarter rounds, ½ cup
1 medium cucumber, thin quarter rounds, 2 cups

Lettuce and tofu salad – Yield: 4 cups.

Dressing: Tofu and umeboshi sauce, 1½ cups, page 182
2 medium scallions, thin rounds, ½ cup
½ small carrot, grated or 4 medium radishes, thin
rounds, ¼ cup
1 small celery stalk, thin quarter rounds, ½ cup
2 cups Romaine lettuce, torn into bite-sized squares

Comments – Toss salad with dressing when the dressing is thick and not easily poured, or when the dressing is boiled or sautéed. Mix dressing first and then add vegetables one kind at a time, with those of least measure first. Try boiled umeboshi dressing with radishes and lettuce; or heated oil and vinegar dressing with red onion, cucumbers, tender yellow squash, and lettuce.

Salad Dressings, Mixed

Procedure – Mix ingredients together. Cream butters, umeboshi paste, or miso with each other first. Then add liquid. Thin until pourable or to desired consistency. Gently toss with salad or serve separately.

Soy sauce dressing – for 4 to 6 cups vegetables. Used in Lettuce, cucumber and sunflower salad, page 164. Yield: ¼ cup.

2 Tbsp soy sauce
2 Tbsp lemon juice or brown rice vinegar

Umeboshi paste dressing – for 8 cups vegetables. Used in Lettuce, radish, avocado salad, page 164. Yield: ½ cup.

1 Tbsp umeboshi paste
4 Tbsp nut or seed butter
2 Tbsp lemon or lime juice or brown rice vinegar
3 to 4 Tbsp water for thinning

Nut butter dressing – for 8 cups vegetables. All purpose salad dressing. Yield: ½ cup.

4 Tbsp nut or seed butter
1 Tbsp light miso or soy sauce
1 Tbsp lemon juice or brown rice vinegar
2 Tbsp water

Tahini dressing – for 8 cups vegetables. All-purpose salad dressing. Yield: ½ cup.

4 Tbsp tahini
1 Tbsp umeboshi vinegar
1 Tbsp lemon juice
2 to 3 Tbsp water

Avocado dressing – for 2 to 3 cups vegetables. Used in Cucumber and avocado salad, page 165. Yield: ¾ cup.

---

1 medium avocado, pitted and mashed, ¾ cup
1 Tbsp lemon juice
1 Tbsp soy sauce

Olive oil and umeboshi vinegar dressing – for 4 to 6 cups vegetables. Used in Azuki bean salad, page 172. All-purpose dressing. Yield: ¼ cup.

---

3 Tbsp olive oil
1 Tbsp umeboshi vinegar

Specialty dressing – for 20 cups vegetables or noodles. All-purpose salad or pasta dressing. Yield: 1¼ cup.

---

12 Tbsp (¾ cup) olive oil
3 Tbsp brown rice vinegar
1 Tbsp balsamic vinegar
1 Tbsp toasted sesame oil
3 Tbsp soy sauce

Comments – Mixed dressings are simple and easy to make. They can be thin or thick, depending on choice of salad. Make thinner when dressing will be served separately. Use fresh, soft ingredients. Variations: add scallions, especially good with nut butter dressings; press garlic through a garlic press, especially good with olive oil dressings; add fresh herbs such as finely chopped parsley, dill, and oregano, good with any of the above recipes, except avocado dressing.

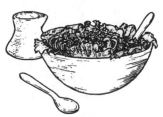

Salad Dressings with Sautéed Onion

Procedure – Heat oil. Sauté onion with sea salt, if used, until transparent. Cover pan. Sauté 5 more minutes over low heat. Remove from heat. Cool 5 minutes. Mix with other dressing ingredients. Let stand 10 minutes. Gently mix with salad.

Onion and lemon dressing – for 8 cups vegetables. Used in Bulgur salad, page 171. Yield: 1½ cups.

---

1 Tbsp light sesame oil or olive oil
1 large onion, finely minced, 2 cups
½ tsp sea salt
1 small lemon, juiced, ¼ cup

Onion and umeboshi paste dressing – for 4 to 6 cups vegetables. Used in Rice salad with cooked vegetables, page 172. Yield: 1½ cups.

---

1 Tbsp light sesame oil or olive oil
1 large onion, finely minced, 2 cups
1 Tbsp umeboshi paste
1 to 2 Tbsp brown rice vinegar or lemon juice

Onion and soy sauce dressing – for 4 to 5 cups vegetables. Used in Rice salad, page 171. Yield: 1½ cups.

---

1 Tbsp light sesame oil or olive oil
1 large onion, finely minced, 2 cups
2 tsp soy sauce
1 Tbsp brown rice vinegar; optional

Comments – These sautéed dressings use onions and especially complement bean, noodle, and grain salads. Cool before mixing with the salad. After mixing the salad, allow to stand 10 to 15 minutes before serving to let flavors mingle. Variations: Sauté garlic with the onion, use more oil, add herbs, or flavor with toasted sesame oil at the end of cooking. Here's a pasta salad to try with this type of cooked dressing: Mix noodles, olives, scallions, boiled snow peas, and optional cooked shrimp with a dressing of light sesame oil, onion, garlic, toasted sesame oil, soy sauce, and brown rice vinegar.

Salad Dressings with Boiled Umeboshi Plums

Procedure – Boil umeboshi plums in the water until soft, 5 to 10 minutes. Remove pits. Mash plums with the cooking water and the other ingredients, using a blender or suribachi. Gently mix with salad.

Umeboshi and scallion dressing – for 8 cups vegetables. Used in Rice and corn salad, page 171. Yield: ½ cup.

4 medium umeboshi plums, whole
¼ cup water
2 medium scallions, thin rounds, ½ cup

Umeboshi and nut butter dressing – for 8 cups vegetables. Used in Cabbage cooked salad, page 102. Yield: 6 tablespoons.

4 medium umeboshi plums, whole
¼ cup water
1 Tbsp nut or seed butter
3 Tbsp lemon juice

Comments – Whole umeboshi plums often need to be softened before pitting and blending. Use more water if plums are drier. Variations: sauté an onion and purée with the boiled plums, or add to the already puréed mixture; mince a red onion and "marinate" in the plum mixture before mixing with the salad; purée red onion with the plums; add dill, basil, mustard, garlic, and oil such as olive oil or light sesame oil. Umeboshi, dill, red onion, and olive oil is a delicious combination. Mix with cooked brown rice, cucumbers, and fresh corn.

Salad Dressings with Heated Oil

Procedure – Lightly heat oil for 15 to 30 seconds. Cool completely, 10 to 12 minutes. Mix well with other ingredients. Gently mix into dish.

Oil and soy sauce dressing – for 3 cups vegetables. Complements spaghetti squash. Yield: 2 tablespoons.

---

    1 Tbsp light sesame oil or olive oil
    1 Tbsp soy sauce

Oil and lemon dressing – for 4 cups vegetables. Complements cooked greens. Yield: about 3 tablespoons.

---

    2 tsp light sesame oil or olive oil
    ¼ tsp sea salt
    2 Tbsp lemon juice

Oil and vinegar dressing – for 5 to 6 cups vegetables. Complements salad. Yield: ¼ cup.

---

    1 Tbsp light sesame oil or olive oil
    ½ tsp sea salt
    3 Tbsp brown rice vinegar

Comments – Heat oil before making dressing to increase flavor. These dressings can be used for salads or cooked vegetables. The oil and soy sauce dressing and the oil and lemon dressing are best when used immediately; the oil and vinegar dressing keeps well and can be made in quantity. Vary these dressings with the addition of garlic, herbs, or spices. For example, sauté garlic briefly and then mix with lemon juice and cooked greens. Or, add dill weed, oregano, granulated onion, pressed garlic, or powdered mustard to the oil and vinegar dressing.

Grain and Bean Salads

Procedure – Prepare dressing. Gently mix ingredients into dressing in the order listed, one kind at a time. Allow flavors to mingle for 30 minutes to 1 hour before serving.

Rice salad – Yield: 5½ cups.

Dressing: Onion and soy sauce dressing, 1½ cups, page 168
½ small carrot, grated, ¼ cup
1 medium cucumber, thin quarter rounds, 2 cups
2 cups cooked brown rice, cooled, page 58 or 68

Bulgur salad – Yield: 8 cups.

Dressing: Onion and lemon dressing, 1½ cups, page 168
½ cup chopped parsley
4 medium scallions, thin rounds, 1 cup
2 medium celery stalks, thin quarter rounds, 1½ cups
4 large radishes, half rounds, ½ cup
4 cups cooked bulgur, cooled, page 59

Rice and corn salad – Serve on lettuce. Garnish as desired. Yield: 6½ cups.

Dressing: Umeboshi and scallion dressing (use 3 plums),
    about 3 Tbsp, page 169
1 small cucumber, thin quarter rounds, 1½ cups
2 ears of corn, cooked and cut off of cob, 2 cups
2 cups cooked brown rice, cooled, page 58 or 68
2 cups lettuce, torn into bite-sized squares
Garnishes: roasted almonds, pages 183-184, nori match-
    sticks, page 134, avocado or tomato wedges, optional

Rice salad with cooked vegetables – See pages 100-102 for boiling vegetables. Yield: 6 cups.

Dressing: Onion and umeboshi paste dressing, 1½ cups, page 168
1 ear of corn, cooked and cut off of cob, 1 cup
1 large carrot, quarter rounds, cook 2 minutes, 1 cup
1 cup broccoli flowerets, 2 inches long, cook 1 minute
2 cups cooked brown rice, cooled, pages 58 or 68

Macaroni salad – Serve on lettuce. Yield: 6 cups.

Dressing: Tofu and tahini sauce, 1½ cups, page 182
2 small celery stalks, thin quarter rounds, 1 cup
1 medium red bell pepper, diced, ¾ cup
2 cups cooked whole wheat macaroni, cooled, page 75
2 cups lettuce, torn into bite-sized squares, 2 cups

Azuki bean salad – Allow minced red onion to sit in dressing 5 minutes before mixing. Yield: 4 cups.

Dressing: Olive oil and umeboshi vinegar dressing, ¼ cup, page 167
½ small red onion, finely minced, ½ cup
1 small celery stalk, thin quarter rounds, ½ cup
1 small carrot, grated, ½ cup
3 cups boiled azuki beans, cooled, page 138

Comments – Grain and bean salads are a refreshing way to prepare a whole meal in one dish, especially in the summer. Try these combinations or invent your own: cooked brown rice, celery, and cucumbers with boiled umeboshi dressing served on lettuce and garnished with roasted walnuts; whole wheat shells, cooked green beans, and scallions with heated oil and vinegar dressing; or any kind of cooked grain, especially quinoa, cooked garbanzo beans, red onion, parsley, celery, carrot, with olive oil and umeboshi vinegar dressing.

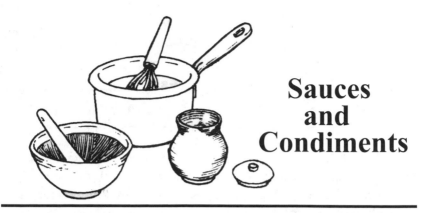

Sauces and Condiments

Use – Sauces, condiments, and dressings add an extra "something" to a meal. Whether it is a simple lemon and soy sauce dressing for tempeh, or an elaborate umeboshi, onion, tahini, dill dip for boiled vegetables, all dressings, sauces, and condiments have this in common: They are the complement to a meal—not the main component.

Flavoring Agents – Dressings, whether cooked or not, usually adorn salads, see previous chapter. Sauces, most often cooked, complement cooked grains, pastas, and vegetables. Condiments are garnishes. Sometimes they are dry, and sometimes they are moist. Most, but not all, dressings, sauces, and condiments are high in fat and salt, and thus are meant to be used as flavoring.

Possibilities – This chapter is a simple introduction to a few types of sauces and condiments using various foods. Many sauces, condiments, and dressings are culinary and are meant to add flavor but some can be used intentionally to balance one's health and condition. There are macrobiotic books available that address these ideas. This book presents preparation methods and variations on the general procedures. For this chapter, feel free to adjust the quantities to suit your own culinary and health needs and to take liberty to invent your own recipes through substitutions and additions.

173

Clear Sauces with Kuzu and Arrowroot

Procedure – Heat oil. Sauté vegetables and seasonings until changed (onion until transparent, mushrooms until condensed). Add half of the water listed. Cover and bring to a boil. Simmer 5 minutes over low heat. For lemon basil sauce, purée in blender, then return to pan. Dissolve arrowroot or kuzu in the other half of the cold water. Add to pan. Simmer until thick and clear, 1 to 2 minutes, stirring constantly. Add soy sauce, or for lemon basil sauce, lemon juice.

Simple clear sauce – Complements wild rice or millet. Yield: 2½ cups.

1 Tbsp light sesame oil or olive oil
1 medium onion, finely minced, 1½ cups
pinch of sea salt
2 cups cold water
2 Tbsp arrowroot or 1 Tbsp kuzu
2 Tbsp soy sauce

Lemon basil sauce – Complements fried fish, burgers, or tempeh. Yield: 2 cups.

1 Tbsp light sesame oil or olive oil
1 medium onion, finely minced, 1½ cups
1 tsp sea salt
1 tsp basil
¼ tsp lemon rind, finely grated
1¾ cups cold water
4 tsp arrowroot or 2 tsp kuzu
¼ cup lemon juice

Mushroom sauce – Good on rice, bulgur, or pasta. Yield: 1 cup.

---

1 Tbsp light sesame oil
¼ pound white mushrooms, sliced, 2 cups
2 medium scallions, thin rounds, ½ cup
thyme leaf, optional
½ tsp sea salt
½ cup water
1 Tbsp arrowroot
1½ to 2 Tbsp soy sauce

Comments – Kuzu and arrowroot are thickening agents and are preferable to cornstarch, which is highly refined. Due to the higher cost of kuzu, I often use arrowroot for culinary use and kuzu for medicinal use, as on page 247. Both cook to a clear consistency in making sauces and can be substituted for each other, using 2 teaspoons arrowroot for 1 teaspoon of kuzu.

Clear sauces are simple to make; just sauté vegetables until tender, thicken with diluted arrowroot or kuzu, and season with soy sauce. Variations: sauté garlic and add to the Simple clear sauce or Mushroom sauce; add toasted sesame oil to the Simple clear sauce or Mushroom sauce; substitute miso for soy sauce in the Mushroom sauce; or simmer with herbs such as dill and oregano in the Lemon basil sauce or thyme leaf in the Mushroom sauce. Other vegetables can be used too, from broccoli to greens. Clear sauces are meant to be simple, more like a simple topping than a main vegetable dish. Make in small amounts for use at one meal and make 5 to 10 minutes before serving.

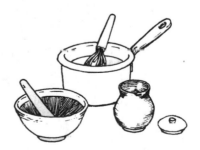

Mixed Sauces with Ginger

Procedure – Grate fresh ginger root on a Japanese or other fine grater. Squeeze out juice. Discard pulp. Mix with other ingredients.

Soy and ginger sauce – Yield: ¼ cup.

1 Tbsp fresh ginger juice
3 to 4 Tbsp soy sauce

Soy and ginger dipping sauce – Yield: ¼ to ½ cup.

1 Tbsp fresh ginger juice
3 to 4 Tbsp soy sauce
1 to 2 Tbsp boiling water or kombu stock, page 124
1 Tbsp toasted sesame oil, optional

Comments – Mixing soy sauce with ginger makes a versatile sauce that is delicious with tofu burgers, polenta, or other fried foods. The Soy and ginger sauce can be used to marinate tempeh before cooking. The Soy and ginger dipping sauce is less salty than the soy and ginger sauce and complements raw or cooked vegetables, or noodles.

Here is a menu suggestion – soba, Soy and ginger dipping sauce with toasted sesame oil, scallions, gomashio, fried fish, avocado, fresh green salad.

Bechamel Sauces with Flour

Procedure – Heat oil. Add flour. Sauté until fragrant, 1 to 2 minutes. Stir constantly to smooth lumps. Remove from heat. Cool completely, 10 to 15 minutes. Mix in half of the amount of cold water listed. Place over medium heat. Slowly add the rest of the cold water, stirring constantly. Use a wire whisk if necessary to smooth lumps. Add sea salt. Cover and bring to a boil. Simmer 20 to 25 minutes over low heat. Stir occasionally. Add water if needed for desired consistency.

Basic bechamel sauce – Yield: 1 cup.

1 Tbsp light sesame oil or olive oil
4 Tbsp whole wheat pastry or other flour
1¼ to 1¾ cups cold water
¼ tsp sea salt

Comments – Bechamel sauce is made by sautéing flour in oil and then simmering with water and salt. Vary the ingredients to make many different sauces. Use more oil for a richer sauce.

Use different flours for variety. Try brown rice flour or sweet brown rice flour for a lighter sauce, or whole wheat flour for a heavier sauce. Corn flour, buckwheat flour, or rye flour can be used also. Sauté the flour longer to make a darker sauce and to increase the flavor.

Simmer with herbs such as parsley, chives, or basil, or sauté the flour with spices such as curry powder or cumin. Add extra seasoning at the end of cooking such as soy sauce, diluted miso, toasted sesame oil, brown rice vinegar, or a dash of maple syrup.

Use water in bechamel sauces or substitute soy or rice milk. Simmer without a cover to thicken; add more liquid to thin.

Serve bechamel sauces over cooked vegetables, noodles, or grains, and garnish with scallions or fresh parsley. Mix bechamel sauces into casseroles or vegetable pie fillings. There are infinite possibilities!

Nut Butter Sauces

Procedure – Cream nut or seed butter with miso or soy sauce, then cream with ¼ cup water. Add scallions, if used. Place over medium heat and add the diluted arrowroot and water. Heat until it boils, 3 to 4 minutes, stirring constantly. It will thicken, so add water or other liquid if needed for desired consistency.

Nut butter sauce – Yield: ½ to ¾ cup.

> 3 Tbsp nut or seed butter
> 1 Tbsp soy sauce or miso
> ¼ cup water
> 2 medium scallions, thin rounds; optional, ½ cup

Nut butter sauce, low fat – Yield: 1¼ to 1¾ cups.

> 3 Tbsp nut or seed butter
> 1 Tbsp soy sauce or miso
> ¼ cup water
> 1 Tbsp arrowroot diluted in ¾ cup water
> 4 medium scallions, thin rounds; optional, 1 cup

Comments – Nut butter sauces are rich and flavorful. They can be made quickly and are best when hot. Serve over noodles or vegetables.

Vary these basic recipes with choice of ingredients. Tahini produces a sauce complementary to most grains, while almond or peanut butter produce a sauce that better complements vegetables. Substitute soy or rice milk for water. Make a light-colored cream sauce with tahini, light miso, and soy milk.

Flavor after sauce boils and thickens; remove from heat and add 1 tablespoon brown rice vinegar, lemon, lime, or orange juice. Peanut butter, miso, and orange juice make a tangy sauce. Add herbs and spices as desired; from simple ginger juice or dill weed in tahini sauce to spicy cayenne in peanut butter sauce.

Chunky Nut Sauces

Procedure – Roast nuts or seeds, page 183 or 184. Chop with a knife if nuts are large or firm. Grind in a blender, food processor, or suribachi until three-fourths of the nuts or seeds are crushed. Add the rest of the ingredients and grind together. Add water, as needed, until creamy and thinned to desired consistency.

Walnut miso – Use as a chunky condiment for rice. Yield: ¾ cup.

    1 cup walnuts
    1 Tbsp dark miso
    1 to 2 Tbsp boiling water for thinning

Walnut sauce with soy sauce – Use as a sauce for mochi or pasta. Yield: 1 cup.

    1 cup walnuts
    1 Tbsp soy sauce
    ½ cup boiling water

Pesto – Yield: 1½ cup.

    ½ cup walnuts
    2 to 4 cloves garlic, pressed through garlic press
    1 bunch basil, 4 cups
    4 to 6 Tbsp olive oil
    2 Tbsp miso or umeboshi paste

Peanut sauce with miso – Yield: ¾ cup.

    1 cup raw peanuts
    1 Tbsp dark miso or soy sauce
    3 Tbsp boiling water

Comments – Sauces made with freshly ground nuts have more texture and taste fresher than sauces made with nut or seed butters. Make thick to use as a spread or make thin to use as a sauce over noodles or grain. Grind nuts completely before mixing or processing with other ingredients.

Vary ingredients for various sauces, using almonds, pumpkin seeds, sunflower seeds, sesame seeds, or other nuts or seeds. Use a dark miso such as soybean or 2-year-old barley miso for a hearty, rich sauce, a light variety such as rice miso for a delicate sauce, or mix as desired. Umeboshi paste or vinegar can be substituted for miso or soy sauce. Add extra ingredients such as freshly squeezed ginger juice, pressed garlic, brown rice vinegar, rice syrup, and herbs as desired. For more information on using a suribachi, see page 42.

Walnut miso can be made for traveling: roast walnuts and grind with miso; cool and pack into container; add water when using.

Here are some ideas for you to try: walnuts, umeboshi paste, and ginger juice; pumpkin seeds, umeboshi vinegar, and rice syrup; sunflower seeds, soy sauce, water, and a dash of brown rice vinegar.

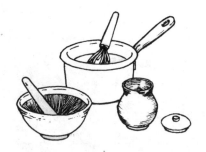

Miso Sauces

Procedure – Heat oil. Add miso. Sauté until fragrant, 1 to 2 minutes, stirring constantly to smooth lumps. Add liquid gradually, thinning to desired consistency. For thin sauce, bring to a boil after adding liquid.

Thick miso sauce – Yield: ¼ cup.

1 Tbsp light sesame oil
3 Tbsp dark miso
1 Tbsp water, lemon, or orange juice

Thin miso sauce – Yield: ½ cup.

1 Tbsp light sesame oil
3 Tbsp dark miso
4 Tbsp water

Comments – Cornellia Aihara called these sauces "oily miso" sauces. Dark miso such as soybean or 2-year-old barley is traditionally used, yet lighter or younger misos can be used. The thick sauce can be used as a spread, especially delicious and beautiful served on rounds of steamed daikon radish or raw cucumber. The thin sauce can be used as a dip for vegetables or a sauce for cooked pasta. For variety, add thin rounds of scallions.

Other variations: sauté finely minced ginger in oil before adding miso; add finely grated lemon or orange peel after adding miso.

Tofu Sauces

Procedure – Boil tofu in water for 5 minutes. Drain and discard water. Blend with other ingredients in a blender or food processor until smooth, thinning to desired consistency. Taste and adjust seasonings.

Tofu and tahini sauce – For 4 to 6 cups pasta or vegetables. Used in Macaroni salad, page 172. Yield: 1½ cups.

½ pound firm tofu, 1-inch cubes, 2 cups
½ cup water
2 Tbsp tahini
2 Tbsp soy sauce or 1 Tbsp miso
½ tsp granulated garlic, optional
2 to 3 Tbsp water, lemon juice, or brown rice vinegar

Tofu and umeboshi sauce – If using umeboshi plums, purée in blender first. Heat oil, add curry powder and cool before mixing. Used in Lettuce and tofu salad, page 165. For 3 to 4 cups pasta or vegetables. Yield: 1½ cups.

½ pound firm tofu, 1-inch cubes, 2 cups
½ cup water
3 to 4 soft umeboshi plums, pitted; or 3 to 4 tsp
    umeboshi paste
2 tsp light sesame oil or olive oil
¼ tsp curry powder, or more
2 Tbsp lemon juice or brown rice vinegar

Comments – Use tofu sauces as spreads, dressings, or sauces, or mix into dishes. Make sauce thick for use as a dip or spread; make thin for use as a topping or ingredient in a dish. Boil the tofu to freshen and make more digestible. For variation, sauté 1 clove of finely minced garlic in the oil, or gently mix thin rounds of scallions or chopped alfalfa sprouts into the blended sauce.

This general procedure is unlimited in variation. Basically tofu is boiled, then blended with a salt source such as soy sauce, miso, or umeboshi; a fat source such as nuts, nut butter, or oil; and a liquid source such as water, lemon juice, soy or rice milk, or vinegar. Add other ingredients as desired: sautéed onion or garlic, dill or fresh basil, curry or cumin. A fun recipe is tofu, umeboshi, almonds, olive oil, garlic, and fresh basil.

Roasted Nuts and Seeds, Oven

Procedure – Place one layer of any kind of nut or seed on a baking sheet. Place in a pre-heated, 350-degree oven. Roast until fragrant, beginning to pop, and browning. Stir occasionally.

> almonds, 12 minutes
> cashews, 7 minutes
> pumpkin seeds, 7 minutes
> raw Spanish peanuts, 12 minutes
> sunflower seeds 10 minutes
> walnuts, 7 minutes

Comments – Roast nuts or seeds in the oven when roasting a large quantity. Stir occasionally as temperatures can vary within the oven. In addition, individual ovens can vary in their heat; these timings are approximate. Watch carefully and remove from oven when seeds and nuts have changed color, before completely browned.

For mixed nuts, roast separately, even if both take the same time. If roasted together, they may not roast uniformly or completely. After roasting, mix while warm.

If desired, add soy sauce after roasting. Place hot roasted nuts or seeds in a bowl. Add 3 or 4 drops soy sauce per ¼ cup nuts or seeds. They will sizzle. Stir to coat. Avoid excess soy sauce as nuts or seeds can become soggy. If this happens, return to oven to dry.

Enjoy roasted nuts or seeds as a snack, as a crunchy topping for noodles, grains, or cooked vegetables, or in baked goods.

Roasted Nuts and Seeds, Top of Stove

Procedure – Place one layer of any kind of nut or seed in a skillet. Dry roast (no oil) over medium heat until fragrant, beginning to pop, and browning. Stir often or shake every 30 seconds. Remove from heat and let stand in hot pan a few extra minutes to complete roasting.

---

almonds, 4 to 5 minutes
cashews, 4 to 5 minutes
pumpkin seeds, 4 to 5 minutes
raw Spanish peanuts, 5 to 6 minutes
sunflower seeds, 4 to 5 minutes
walnuts, 4 to 5 minutes
sesame seeds (wash and drain before roasting),
    4 to 5 minutes

Comments – Roast nuts or seeds on top of the stove when roasting a small amount. Nuts and seeds have close contact with the heat so stir often so they roast uniformly. Nuts and seeds are done when they have changed flavor; they don't have to brown completely. Stand in the pan for extra time to receive the heat of the pan and complete roasting the insides without over-browning the outsides. Let larger nuts remain in the pan longer than smaller seeds. If the pan is already hot, roasting may be faster than the times specified.

If desired, add soy sauce after roasting. Place hot nuts or seeds in a bowl. Add 3 or 4 drops of soy sauce per ¼ cup nuts or seeds. They will sizzle. Stir to coat. Avoid excess soy sauce as nuts or seeds can become soggy. If this happens, return to pan to dry.

Roasted Sesame Seeds, Covered Skillet

Procedure – Wash seeds and drain. Place one very thin layer of seeds, 2 to 3 tablespoons, in a lightweight, dry skillet (no oil). Cover. Roast over medium heat. Shake pan every 5 to 10 seconds. Seeds will pop, smell fragrant, and brown. The first batch will roast in 4 to 5 minutes; subsequent batches will roast quicker as the pan becomes hotter. When done, seeds will be easy to crush between two fingers. Remove and continue for remaining seeds, roasting in small batches.

Roasted sesame seeds

1 cup whole, brown sesame seeds

Comments – Roast small amounts of sesame seeds in a covered skillet to thoroughly roast seeds. They have more contact with the heat than when roasted in large amounts. The cover keeps the popping seeds and heat inside. Use a small, lightweight skillet for ease in handling.

This method is preferred for sesame seeds that will be used in condiments, page 186. If the seeds will be added to dough, they can be roasted by the top-of-the stove method as they will roast again when baked. Each method takes the same amount of time overall to roast the same quantity of seeds; one cup of seeds will take about 15 minutes to roast by either method.

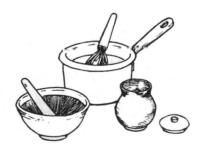

Roasted Sesame Seed Condiments

Procedure – Place sea salt, if used, in a dry skillet (no oil) and roast over medium heat for one minute, stirring constantly. Roast wakame if used, page 134. Place hot wakame or sea salt in suribachi. Grind to a fine powder. Roast sesame seeds by the covered skillet method, page 185. Add to suribachi and grind gently until three-fourths of the seeds are crushed.

Sesame seed salt (gomashio) – Yield: 1½ cups.

1 Tbsp sea salt
1 cup whole, brown sesame seeds

Sesame seed wakame condiment – Yield: 1½ cups.

3 strips wakame, will make about 2 Tbsp powder
1 cup whole, brown sesame seeds

Comments – Gomashio is a traditional Japanese condiment complementary to most grains, noodles, vegetables, and salads commonly used in macrobiotic cooking. The proportion of sea salt to seeds is 1 to 16 and can be adjusted. Use wakame in place of sea salt for a low-salt condiment.

A suribachi, see page 42, is preferred over a blender to make these condiments as a suribachi gently crushes the seeds and allows the oil to coat the sea salt while a blender merely cuts the seeds.

Roast the sea salt before making gomashio to dry and to make it easier to grind. These condiments will keep for up to 1 month at room temperature.

Other sesame seed condiments can be made by substituting dark miso or umeboshi for the sea salt. Grind roasted sesame seeds completely first. Use 1 teaspoon miso, 1 pitted umeboshi plum, or 1 teaspoon umeboshi paste per ¼ cup seeds.

Spreads

Procedure – For nut butter spread, cream all ingredients together. For hummus, drain beans and reserve water. Process garlic in food processor, then add rest of ingredients except parsley and process until smooth. Fold in parsley.

Nut butter spread – Yield: ½ cup.

¼ cup nut or seed butter
2 tsp miso or soy sauce
2 Tbsp water
1 scallion, chopped, 2 Tbsp

Quick hummus – Yield: 1¼ cup.

1½ cups cooked garbanzo beans, drained, 15 oz can
1 clove garlic, ½ tsp
1 Tbsp tahini
4 to 5 tsp lemon juice
sea salt to taste, if beans are unsalted
2 to 3 Tbsp reserved bean water
1 Tbsp minced parsley

Comments – These two spreads are easy and quick to prepare. For nut butter spread, use tahini, peanut butter, almond butter, or others. Add grated carrot, parsley, or chopped alfalfa sprouts for variety.

The quick hummus is a classic recipe. Substitute other beans as desired.

Pickles and Pressed Salads

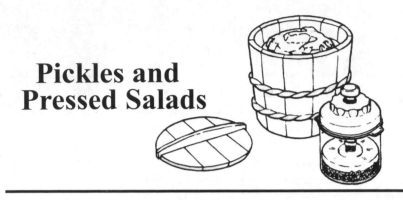

Fermentation – Pickles are a fermented food, a necessary addition to a grain-based diet. Grains are hearty and substantial, requiring adequate digestion. Pickles are a digestive aid. Through fermentation, bacteria thrive, and through natural pickling techniques, healthy bacteria are encouraged. Fermentation provides enzymes and vitamins to the intestinal flora and strengthens the digestive tract.

Natural pickling all year around – Pickles are made with simple ingredients: vegetables, good quality sea salt or other salt source, water, and time. Distilled white vinegar, crude iodized salt, and canning are avoided. Pickles are made in small batches and can be made in any season. Pickle at room temperature. In summer, pickling is faster because bacteria are more active.

Duration of pickling – Pickling can be done in a short time such as 1 to 2 hours for quick pressed salads, or in a long time such as 2 weeks for sauerkraut. Generally, pickles are done when they change color and flavor, and when the sea salt has permeated them. Pressed salads are done when they have condensed and absorbed some sea salt, but are still crisp.

Vegetables – Use clean, blemish-free vegetables. Young crisp vegetables make better pickles than older vegetables. Wash and air-dry vegetables before starting pickles to reduce excess moisture. Vegetables that are at room temperature produce better pickles than vegetables right out of the refrigerator, so let vegetables stand 1 hour at room temperature before pickling.

Sea Salt – Sea salt helps keep unfriendly bacteria in check. It permeates the vegetables, adding flavor and preserving them. Sea salt also makes the pickles alkaline-forming so they complement acid-forming grains. For pickles made in bran or brine, the longer the pickles stay in the medium, the more salty they become. Use the best quality sea salt you can find.

Pressed salads – Pressed salads are a cross between raw salads and pickles. They are included in this chapter because they use the same techniques as pickles. Vegetables are mixed with sea salt or brine and pressed like pickles but stand for less time so they remain crunchy like salads. Pressed salads are made with less sea salt than pickles. While pickles are served in small amounts, pressed salads can be served in quantities closer to raw salad. In addition, make small quantities of pressed salads and use when made; they are best when fresh.

Containers – Pickle in a deep container that will not leak. While vegetables are pickling, they must be surrounded completely by the medium; contact with air can cause spoiling. Three types of pickle containers are described and illustrated. Take special care to clean all equipment that will come in contact with the food or brine. Be as hygienic as possible. Wash equipment and rinse well in hot water, then scald with boiling water.

Japanese pickle press – A pickle press is a special tool, usually made of plastic, to make pickles through pressure. Many sizes are available; a common size holds about 2½ quarts. The lid screws on and has an adjustable spring, which applies pressure to a disc. The pressure can be adjusted for different types of pickles; for example, strong pressure for pressed pickles and light pressure for brine pickles.

Crock with a weighted plate – This "press" can be assembled from common kitchen utensils. Ingredients are packed into a large container such as a crock or a large bowl made of ceramic or glass. A plate that fits inside the container without touching the sides is placed on top of the ingredients. A heavy weight, like a gallon jar of water or a heavy rock, may be put on the plate to apply a lot of pressure, as when making pressed pickles. A medium weight, like a small jar of water or a light rock, may be put on the plate to apply just enough pressure to keep the vegetables under the liquid, as when making brine pickles. The weight may be left off so there is only the pressure from the plate, as when making bran pickles. A clean cloth is placed over the entire container to keep out dust.

Two jars – Use two jars when pickling vegetables in brine. The small jar fits inside the large jar and keeps the vegetables submerged. To use, pack vegetables into a gallon jar. Cover with brine. Slip a plastic lid from a storage container inside the jar. Rest lid on top of the vegetables. (This lid will keep all the vegetables down.) Fit the small jar into the large jar so it rests on the plastic lid. Screw on the lid of the large jar. If the lid of the large jar does not hold down the small jar, fill the small jar with water to apply enough weight to keep the vegetables submerged.

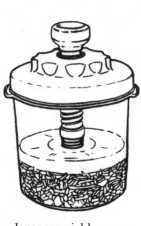

Japanese pickle press

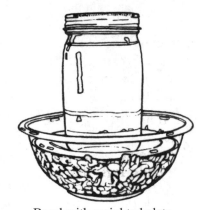

Bowl with weighted plate

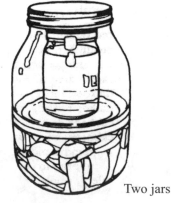

Two jars

Salt Brine Pickles and Pressed Salads

Procedure – Boil water and sea salt until the salt has dissolved. Cool completely. Wash all vegetables and air-dry completely. Clean and scald equipment for making pickles, and air-dry. Pack vegetables tightly in container. Cover vegetables completely with the brine. Apply enough weight to keep vegetables submerged. Ferment or press at room temperature for the time indicated. Remove from brine when serving.

Cucumber dill pickles – Ferment 3 to 4 days. Yield: 2½ quarts.

brine of 5 cups water and 10 tsp sea salt
20 three-inch pickling cucumbers, whole, or 15 five-inch
1 large onion, large crescents, 2 cups
1 clove garlic, thinly sliced; ½ tsp black peppercorns;
    2 bay leaves, optional
2 sprigs fresh dill, whole, or 1 tsp dill seed

Cabbage, cucumber, and carrot pressed salad – Press 4 to 5 hours. Yield: 5 cups.

brine of 1 cup water and 1 tsp sea salt
1 small cabbage (core removed), shredded, 4 cups
1 medium cucumber, thin quarter rounds, 2 cups
½ small carrot, grated, ¼ cup

Lettuce and carrot pressed salad – Press 1 to 2 hours. Yield: 3½ cups.

brine of 1 cup water and 1 tsp sea salt
4 cups Romaine lettuce, shredded, use inner white parts
2 medium scallions, thin rounds, ½ cup
½ small carrot, grated, ¼ cup

Comments – Making brine pickles is perhaps the easiest and most familiar of the pickling techniques covered in this book. It works beautifully with pickling cucumbers, but root vegetables also pickle well. Almost any vegetable can be pickled with this procedure; make sure to keep vegetables submerged while pickling. Any of the containers described on pages 189-190 can be used with good results.

The brine used for making pickles contains 2 teaspoons sea salt per 1 cup water. The brine used for making pressed salads contains 1 teaspoon sea salt per 1 cup water. Use enough brine to cover the vegetables by ¼ inch, and enough weight to keep the vegetables submerged. As the vegetables pickle they will shrink and release some water, so the amount of liquid will increase.

Watch carefully for healthy signs of fermentation—rising bubbles and a good smell. The bubbles will be white the first day and may darken the next. If there are no bubbles after 24 hours, the room is too cool. Move the pickles into a warmer place or even into the sun to speed fermentation. If fermentation is too active such as bubbles overflowing the container, move to a cooler place. Pickles should smell pleasant. If there is a drastic change in color or smell, skim to remove bubbles and move to a cooler place.

Fermentation is complete in 3 to 4 days for cucumbers and most root vegetables. After 3 days check pickles by tasting. Pickles are done when the flavor has changed and the color has deepened.

Pickles will keep about 2 months in the refrigerator and will continue to ferment somewhat after the initial fermentation. Some pickles may turn soft, especially if older vegetables were used. If white mold occurs while pickling, the brine does not have enough salt or the vegetables were not fresh. If mold occurs while pickles are in the refrigerator, the pickles are becoming too old.

Pressed salads are easy to make with salt brine. Use a Japanese pickle press or a bowl with a weight. Press cabbage salads longer, up to 24 hours, for a slightly pickled salad.

Soy Sauce Brine Pickles and Pressed Salads

Procedure – Bring soy sauce and water to a boil. Cool completely. Clean and scald container when making pickles. Pack washed and dried vegetables tightly in container. Cover with the brine. Weight to keep the vegetables submerged. Ferment or press at room temperature for the time indicated. Remove from brine when serving.

Onion, radish, and carrot pickles – Ferment 3 to 4 days. Yield: 2 cups.

brine of ¾ cup soy sauce and 1½ cups water (enough for
   3 cups cut vegetables)
1 large onion, large crescents, 2 cups
4 medium red radishes, thick rounds, ¼ cup
1 medium carrot, thin diagonals, ¾ cup

Daikon pickles – Ferment 3 to 4 days. Yield: 3 cups.

brine of 1 cup soy sauce and 2 cups water
1 medium daikon radish, "logs," thin half rounds, or thin
   "paper-cut" slices, 4 cups

Lettuce, cucumber, and scallion pressed salad – Press 1 to 2 hours. Yield: 4 cups.

brine of 2 Tbsp soy sauce and ½ cup water
4 cups shredded Romaine lettuce, inner white part
2 medium scallions, thin rounds, ½ cup
1 medium cucumber, thin quarter rounds, 2 cups

Comments – Root and cut vegetables make delicious soy sauce pickles. Vegetables will absorb color, but are tasty. Any of the containers described on pages 189-190 can be used with good results. Vegetables need to be kept under the brine but don't need a lot of pressure.

The brine used for making soy sauce pickles contains 2 parts water to 1 part soy sauce. It is important to use high-quality unpasteurized soy sauce for these pickles for best flavor and health benefits. Boiling the brine prevents molding. Use enough brine to cover vegetables; as they pickle, they will shrink and release water, which will increase the amount of liquid. After all the pickles have been eaten, the brine can be used for second and third batches of pickles. For an original brine of ½ cup soy sauce and 1 cup water, bring used brine to a boil, remove from heat, then add ¼ cup soy sauce. Cover completely and proceed with the pickling procedure.

Pickles will keep about 2 months in the refrigerator where they will continue to pickle and become more flavorful. After the initial fermentation they will be crunchy, but in 10 days, they will soften

Salads pressed in soy sauce brine are delicious. It is my favorite way to prepare pressed salad. Vegetables will keep their own colors because they are pressed for a short time. Use 1 part soy sauce to 3 to 4 parts water for brine. You can use the brine without boiling; a salad pressed a short time will not mold. Use a pickle press or bowl with a weight to make salad pressed in soy sauce brine.

Try other root vegetables to make pickles, such as turnips or rutabagas. Use singly or in combination with onion. Cabbage, carrots, and radishes make good pressed salads, too.

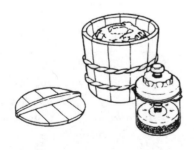

Pressed Pickles and Salads

Procedure – Mix thinly sliced vegetables with sea salt thoroughly scrunching vegetables by hand to soften them. If you have a suribachi, use it to mix the vegetables and sea salt, kneading them against the sides of the suribachi. If your suribachi is small, mix proportional amounts of vegetables and sea salt in quantities that will fit.

Pack tightly into a Japanese pickle press. If using bay leaves, place 2 cups of the vegetable and sea salt mixture in the press and place a small bay leaf on top. Repeat layers ending with a bay leaf on top. Place cover on the press, screw down, and press strongly. Water from the vegetables will rise to cover them. Ferment or press at room temperature for the time indicated. Bubbles will arise in 24 to 30 hours. When serving, remove liquid from portion to be served.

Pressed cabbage pickles – Ferment 3 to 4 days. Yield: 5½ cups.

1 large cabbage (core removed), shredded, 15 cups
1 tsp sea salt per 4 cups shredded cabbage
bay leaves, optional

Pressed lettuce and cucumber salad – Press 1 to 2 hours. Yield: 3½ cups.

4 cups shredded Romaine lettuce, white inner parts
1 medium cucumber, thin quarter rounds, 2 cups
1 tsp sea salt

Pressed Chinese cabbage and radish salad – Press 4 to 5 hours. Yield: 1¾ cups.

6 Chinese cabbage leaves, shredded, 2½ cups
4 large radishes, thin rounds, ½ cup
½ tsp sea salt

Pressed Chinese cabbage pickles – Ferment 3 to 4 days. Yield: 5½ cups.

---

1 large Chinese cabbage
   core, finely minced
   leaves, shredded thinly, 15 cups
1 tsp sea salt per 4 cups shredded cabbage
2 to 3 Tbsp ginger root, finely minced, optional

Comments – Pressing vegetables with sea salt works best for watery vegetables like cabbage, radishes, and cucumbers. Pressure and sea salt draw out water from the vegetables. Dense root vegetables like carrots and turnips have less water and should be used in combination with cabbage rather than alone.

This procedure is designed to use a minimal amount of sea salt and features a suribachi and a Japanese pickle press. A suribachi softens the vegetables when mixing so the sea salt permeates easily. A Japanese pickle press gives the best results for this procedure because it applies strong pressure, which draws out water.

If you don't have a suribachi, mix vegetables and sea salt thoroughly by hand. If you don't have a Japanese pickle press, use a bowl with a weight. Increase the amount of sea salt to 2 teaspoons sea salt per 4 cups shredded vegetables. Mix vegetables and sea salt, then pack into a bowl and place a plate on top of the vegetables. Weight with a heavy rock or bottle of water. Cover with a clean cloth, page 190.

Check to make sure the liquid is rising to cover the vegetables. For pickles, if liquid doesn't cover the vegetables after 4 hours, add salted brine to cover (2 teaspoons sea salt per 1 cup water). If liquid doesn't rise to cover the vegetables, it could be from too little salt; too little pressure; vegetables and salt mixed inadequately; or vegetables being too cold at the start. If the liquid did rise and mold developed, too little salt was used. Vegetables must be covered with liquid or they may spoil.

Pressed pickles will keep for up to 2 months. After the initial fermentation of 3 to 4 days, pack tightly into clean jars and refrigerate to slow down the fermentation. At first, the pickles will be slightly crisp, but they will soften after 5 days, and become more flavorful.

An alternate method to making pressed salads is to layer shredded vegetables and sea salt in a bowl. Increase sea salt to 3 teaspoons per 4 cups vegetables. Weight as above. When water rises, remove the weight, rinse salad to remove excess sea salt, and serve.

Try other combinations such as cabbage mixed with cucumbers or scallions, or daikon radish cut into matchsticks for pickles. Use lettuce or cabbage alone, or with radishes, scallions, turnips, or carrots for pressed salads.

Quick Pickles

Use – These pickles are made quickly using umeboshi vinegar, sea salt, or brown rice vinegar and soy sauce for fermentation. The cucumber "pickle" makes a fresh addition to summer menus.

Red radish pickles – Slice red radishes into thin rounds and mix with umeboshi vinegar at a proportion of 1 to 2 drops per slice, or ½ teaspoon umeboshi vinegar for ½ cup sliced radishes. These can be mixed and served or allowed to stand for 1 to 2 hours.

Cucumber quick pickles – Slice cucumbers into thin rounds, half or quarter rounds. Mix with ¼ teaspoon sea salt per medium cucumber (2 cups). Sea salt draws out moisture from the cucumbers. These can be mixed and served or allowed to stand for up to 1 hour before serving.

Jicama light pickle – Mix 2 tablespoons umeboshi vinegar and 2 teaspoons olive oil. Slice 2 cups jicama into matchsticks and marinate 30 minutes or longer.

Brown rice vinegar and soy sauce quick pickles – Mix 1 tablespoon brown rice vinegar and 1 tablespoon soy sauce. Slice ½ cup of daikon radish, onion, red radish, turnip, or jicama, and marinate 1 hour or longer.

Rice Bran Pickles (Nuka Pickles)

Procedure – Bran mixture: Roast rice bran and sea salt together in a dry pan (no oil) until fragrant, about 15 minutes. Stir often to prevent burning and to smooth out lumps. Cover and cool completely.

Pickling: Wash vegetables and drain until dry. Cut or leave whole as directed. Use a wide-mouth crock or jar, at least a 2-quart size. Press a one-inch layer of the bran mixture in the bottom of the container. Place a layer of vegetables on top so they do not touch each other. Cover completely with bran mixture, press down. Repeat layers, ending with bran mixture. Press down firmly. Place a small flat plate or board on bran. Cover container with a cloth. Remove pickles from the container after the indicated time, and brush off bran. If not serving immediately, store in a covered container in the refrigerator. Don't wash until immediately before slicing. When ready to serve, wash off remaining bran, pat dry, and slice into bite-sized pieces such as half-rounds, "logs," thin "paper-cut" slices, or diagonals.

Bran mixture

1 cup sea salt per 5 cups rice bran

Vegetables – Use individually or in combination.

red radish, whole – 8 to 12 hours
cucumber, peeled, 2-inch rounds – 8 to 12 hours
cucumber, peeled, whole – 12 to 18 hours
radish greens, whole – 8 to 12 hours
daikon radish, 2-inch rounds – 12 to 18 hours
daikon radish, whole (1½-inch diameter) – 24 to 30 hours
cabbage, leaf – 8 to 12 hours
cabbage, whole and cored – 12 hours for the outer leaves;
    remove pickled outer leaves and replace cabbage head
    in bran to continue pickling, 12 hours each time
celery, whole or halved – 8 to 12 hours
bok choy, whole or halved – 8 to 12 hours

Comments – This recipe was developed by Cornellia Aihara and is included for those who want to try to make these authentic Japanese pickles. Nuka means rice bran in Japanese. In Japan, nuka pickle barrels are kept for many years. Pickles are made often, and the wet mixture is stirred daily to ensure that it will last. Rice bran produces a fermentation for vegetables that is especially complementary for grains. The bran is dry and very salty, so it will keep well. If you can't find rice bran, substitute wheat bran.

Vegetables are pickled in large pieces because small pieces absorb too much salt, shrink, and lose their shape. Pickle a small amount of vegetables at a time and remove from the pickling container after the initial fermentation period. Pickles are done when they shrink and change color and the sea salt has permeated them. After removing from the bran, the vegetables will pickle somewhat until they are washed. Use after washing as washed pickles spoil easily.

The new bran mixture is dry, and the first few batches will be more salty. At first, pickle only a few vegetables at a time such as 4 red radishes, and use within 2 days. In time, the bran will soften from the juices drawn out from the vegetables, and the pickles will taste less salty. When the mixture becomes very wet, roast more bran with sea salt and mix completely into the old bran mixture.

Keep mixture at room temperature in a cool place. Tend daily, especially as the mixture becomes more wet, mixing top to bottom. Before placing vegetables in the bran, remove bran from container and mix well. Then layer bran, vegetables, bran. If you must be away, the bran mixture will keep for about one month untended: Remove all vegetables, press down the bran and sprinkle 1 tablespoon dry sea salt per 5 to 6 cups of bran on top. The mixture may be refrigerated in hot weather. Remove any mold that develops on the bran. If the bran smells good, it can still be used.

A large container can be used to pickle many vegetables. A five gallon crock with 15 to 20 cups of bran works well for pickling whole vegetables such as daikon or cabbage and when making pickles for many people on a daily basis.

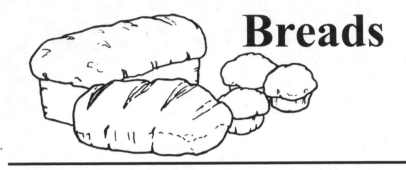

Breads

Flour – Breads made from whole grain flours are nutritive and substantial. Full-bodied and full-flavored, yeasted or naturally-leavened, homemade bread provides familiarity in a grain-based diet.

Whole wheat flour is the basic ingredient in bread. Wheat produces gluten—a necessary substance that traps the expanding yeast and makes the bread rise. Spelt and kamut flours can be substituted and provide adequate gluten. Rye flour, cornmeal, and buckwheat flour have less gluten and are usually used in combination with whole wheat flour. Loaf breads require at least 50 percent whole wheat (spelt or kamut) flour for proper leavening. Quick breads such as biscuits or pancakes can be made with any flour alone or with less percentage of whole wheat flour.

Leavening – Leaven is used to add air to bread so it is more digestible and edible. Customarily, baker's yeast is used for breads; baking powder is used in quick breads. Both are predictable and provide "fast" leavening. Both are useful when learning to bake breads and when serving guests. Use quality products: purchase bulk dry baker's yeast and aluminum-free baking powder from a natural food store.

Some people react to baker's yeast and baking powder, however, and prefer natural leavening. Natural leavening relies on airborne yeasts. The air contains beneficial bacteria and yeasts, and during lengthy contact with the dough these microbes become active and cause the dough to rise.

Sourdough – True "sourdough" bread uses a starter and is a wonderful way to make bread. For years I have used starter to make sourdough bread and while I endorse it completely, it is beyond the scope of this book, mainly because it is vital to have a workable and live starter. I have had the most success after receiving a starter from a more experienced baker rather than trying to "grow" my own. If you ever have a chance to take a class on sourdough bread baking and to obtain your own starter, seize the opportunity. This book covers naturally-leavened breads that resemble the true sourdough but will be more dense.

Ingredients – All ingredients, except the first warm water for baker's yeast, should be used at room temperature. Cold ingredients can halt the leavening time. Hot ingredients can neutralize the leavening power. Leftovers such as noodle water, cooked grains, fruits, and vegetables can be used successfully when at room temperature.

Oil and salt – Oil may be added to dough to give a rich texture and flavor, see pages 16-17. Salt enhances the flavor and helps maintain acid-alkaline balance. It toughens the gluten in kneaded breads, giving the bread more texture and elasticity for rising. Salt also helps control the growth of unwanted yeasts. Use a natural sea salt for baking.

Proportion of flour to water – A higher proportion of flour to water makes a stiffer dough. Loaf breads contain more flour than batter breads and biscuits. Since different flours absorb different amounts of water, keep the end result in mind while mixing. For example, kneaded loaf doughs should be firm and not sticky; biscuit doughs should be thick and wet; pancake batter should be thin and pourable.

Kneading – Dough for loaf bread is kneaded to develop gluten, which gives dough its rising ability. Knead for 10 to 15 minutes until the dough is smooth and no longer sticky. Use a lightly floured surface or a bowl twice the size of the dough and add flour in small increments while kneading.

Kneading stretches the dough and involves a whole-body movement. Basically, push the dough away from you with the heels of the hands, turn it one quarter turn, and pick up the far edge, folding it towards you. Push it away again, turn, fold, repeat. To make kneading in a bowl easier, place the bowl on the floor, kneel, and sit on your heels. Raise your body up and back while pulling and folding. Lower your body and lean forward while pushing dough. This movement prevents aching shoulders.

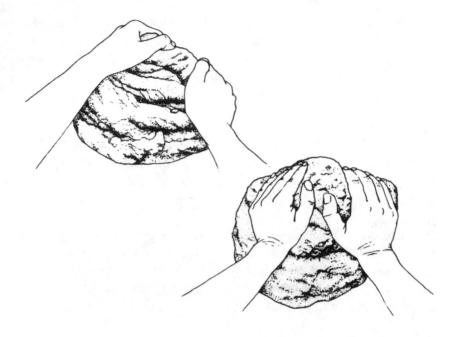

Rising or resting dough – Bake biscuits and muffins made with baking powder immediately. Other kinds of breads and doughs need time to rise. Kneaded loaf breads made with baker's yeast rise over a period of hours. Naturally-leavened doughs rise longer, even overnight, to have contact with airborne yeasts. Check dough while rising; let it rise until it has expanded and smells pleasant. The rising time will vary. In the summer, yeasted doughs will rise in 2 to 4 hours and naturally-leavened ones in 8 to 10 hours. In the winter, allow 6 to 8 hours for yeasted doughs and up to 24 hours for naturally-leavened ones.

Naturally-leavened batter breads, unleavened biscuits, muffins, and pancakes should rest 15 minutes to 4 hours to allow the ingredients to mix and swell. Batter breads can be set in the sun to rise.

During the time of rising or resting, cover bowl with a damp cloth to prevent dough from drying out or crusting.

Forming the loaves – After the dough has risen, cut dough with a table knife and form it into loaf shapes. Smooth creases and lines for an even crust. Fit dough into oiled bread pans, about three-quarters full, and gently press into corners as needed.

Place filled bread pans in a warm oven for 1 hour to rise and warm before baking. An oven with a pilot light provides a good temperature. If your oven has no pilot light or is electric, heat the oven for a few minutes, turn it off, and place bread inside. Remove bread while preheating oven to baking temperature.

Oiling pans – Oil pans before filling. Use coconut oil or butter if desired. See pages 16-17, or use parchment paper to line baking sheets.

Baking – Slash tops with a sharp knife, making one or two ½-inch-deep, lengthwise cuts to allow the bread to expand while baking and to avoid cracking. Bake in a preheated oven until the bottoms are browned. Loaf breads will produce a hollow sound when tapped on the bottom.

Cooling – Bread tastes delicious when hot from the oven but it can be gummy and hard to digest. Let breads cool completely before slicing and eating. The cooling-off time is actually a time for the bread to finish baking. Loaf breads take at least an hour to cool, while biscuits or muffins take 10 minutes. Remove from baking pans to a rack to cool.

Problems – Success in bread baking requires using a recipe over and over to learn how your unique factors such as kind of flour, size of pans, and oven temperature work together. If the dough doesn't rise, either it is too cold, or the yeast is inactive. Set in a warmer place and let rise longer; up to 24 hours for naturally-leavened bread and up to 12 hours for yeasted ones. If, after baking, the crust is too hard, the oven heat was too hot, or the cooking time too long. Steam to soften. If bread sticks to the pans, the pans were oiled too lightly; use these chunks of bread for dipping into soup.

Loaf Breads, Naturally Leavened

Procedure – Place all ingredients except flour into a bowl. Mix well until smooth and without lumps, using a wire whisk if necessary. Add whole wheat flour by the cupful until you can no longer stir it. Add more whole wheat flour, mixing by hand, until the dough is no longer sticky. Knead until smooth, 10 to 15 minutes adding small amounts of flour as necessary. Cover bowl with a damp cloth. Place in a warm spot. Let rise until the dough has expanded, but still smells sweet; 8 to 10 hours in hot weather; up to 24 hours in cold weather. Form into loaves. Place into oiled loaf pans. Let rise 1 hour in a warm oven. Remove from oven. Slit tops. Preheat oven to 350 degrees. Bake for 1 to 1½ hours, depending on size of leaves.

Wheat bread – 3 small loaves.

---

    4 cups water
    1½ tsp sea salt
    10 to 12 cups whole wheat flour

Cooked grain bread – 3 small loaves.

---

    2 cups cooled, cooked grain
    4 cups water
    1½ tsp sea salt (assuming grain was cooked with salt)
    10 to 12 cups whole wheat flour

Comments – Cooked grain bread is the classic "Ohsawa" bread; thick, dense, and chewy. It is a great way to use leftover rice. Variations: substitute 4 cups rye flour, or 1 cup buckwheat flour and 3 cups cornmeal for 4 of the cups of whole wheat flour; mix cooked grains and flours such as cooked barley with wheat flour, or cooked rice with cornmeal and wheat flours. Use at least 50 percent whole wheat flour and add the flour of smallest quantity first. Or, use leftover noodle water or add raisins or roasted nuts. Slice thin and chew well.

Loaf Breads, Yeasted

Procedure – Soften baker's yeast in ½ cup warm water. Add the 2 tablespoons of flour. Stand 10 to 15 minutes in a warm place until bubbly. Add the rest of the warm water, oil, and salt. Mix well. Add whole wheat flour by the cupful until you can no longer stir it. Add more whole wheat flour, mixing by hand, until the dough is no longer sticky. Knead until smooth, 10 to 15 minutes, adding small amounts of flour as necessary. Cover bowl with a damp cloth. Place in a warm spot. Let rise until the dough has expanded, but still smells sweet: 2 to 4 hours in hot weather; 6 to 8 hours in cold weather. Form into leaves. Place into oiled loaf pans. Let rise 1 hour in a warm oven. Remove from oven. Slit tops. Preheat oven to 350 degrees. Bake for 1 to 1¼ hours, depending on the size of the loaves.

Yeasted bread – 4 small loaves or 3 large loaves.

> 1 Tbsp dry baker's yeast
> ½ cup warm water (110 to 115 degrees)
> 2 Tbsp whole wheat, spelt, or kamut flour
> 5 cups warm water
> ¼ cup coconut oil, melted, optional
> 2 tsp sea salt
> 12 to 14 cups whole wheat, spelt, or kamut flour

Comments – Yeasted bread rises in less time than naturally-leavened bread and is a lighter bread, wonderful for guests and holidays. Spelt or kamut flours can be used instead of whole wheat flour and produce loaves similar in flavor and texture to whole wheat. Variations: combine flours with whole wheat flour such as 4 cups rye flour; 4 cups rolled oats; or 2 cups rye flour and 2 cups cornmeal. Make sure loaf contains at least 50 percent whole wheat, kamut, or spelt flour. Add roasted nuts or dried fruits when forming the loaves after the dough has risen. Add cooked puréed vegetables such as squash or carrots to liquid for a vegetable bread.

Batter Breads, Naturally Leavened

Procedure – Mix water, sea salt, and grain, if used, separating the kernels. Add flour and mix until the dough is moist and thick. Beat well. Cover the bowl with a damp cloth. Place in a warm spot. Let rise until the dough is bubbly but still smells sweet: 3 to 4 hours in direct sunlight; 6 to 8 hours indoors in hot weather; up to 12 hours in cold weather. Pour into a well-oiled baking pan. Bake 1¼ hours at 350 degrees.

Cornmeal batter bread – 9″ x 13″ pan.

4 cups water
½ tsp sea salt
1 cup cooled cooked rice, optional
2½ cups cornmeal
2½ to 3 cups whole wheat flour

Comments – Batter bread is easier to make than kneaded bread. The dough is moist and produces a soft bread. Cornbread is very good made by this method, especially when it rises in the sun. A 9- x 13-inch baking pan works well, but loaf pans or muffin tins can be used, too. Oil pans well so bread doesn't stick.

This recipe turns out well with almost any variation. Even the proportions can be changed to more water or flour. I often use leftover grain or water from cooking noodles with this recipe. Other variations include: beat 1 egg and mix into the dough just before filling the pan; substitute soy or rice milk for water; add nuts or raisins before filling pan.

Muffins, Unleavened

Procedure – Mix water, oil, and salt. Add flour(s) and mix thoroughly with a wooden spoon. Batter should be runny. Let the batter rest 20 to 30 minutes. Batter will thicken. Fill heated, well-oiled muffin tins. Bake 30 to 40 minutes at 400 degrees.

Whole wheat muffins – 12 muffins.

---

2 cups water
1 Tbsp coconut oil, melted
¼ tsp sea salt
2½ cups whole wheat pastry flour
2 Tbsp arrowroot powder or brown rice flour

Buckwheat muffins – 12 muffins.

---

2 cups water
1 Tbsp coconut oil, melted
¼ tsp sea salt
1½ cups buckwheat flour
1 cup whole wheat pastry flour

Comments – These recipes are optimal for anyone desiring baked goods without baking powder, soda, or yeast. For best results, use a well-oiled muffin tin, see pages 16-17; paper liners do not work well.

Muffins are moist. The batter is thin and also can be used to make pancakes. For variety use different flours such as cornmeal, rye flour, or barley flour, alone or in combination. Substitute soymilk, rice milk, or water leftover from cooking noodles for water. Add eggs, raisins, or nuts to the batter right before filling tins.

Muffins can be filled with cooked vegetables or fruit. Spoon tins one-third full of batter; add 1 tablespoon filling; spoon batter to top of tin. Try cooked mashed winter squash or sweet potatoes in the whole wheat muffins, or apple butter or raspberry jam in the buckwheat muffins.

Biscuits, Unleavened

Procedure – Mix water, oil, and salt. Add flour(s) and rolled oats, if used. Mix thoroughly with a wooden spoon. Batter should be wet. Let batter thicken 20 to 30 minutes so it holds its shape when spooned onto a well-oiled baking sheet. Bake 35 to 40 minutes at 350 degrees.

Cornmeal biscuits – 14 biscuits.

1½ cups water
2 Tbsp coconut oil, melted
¼ tsp sea salt
1½ cups cornmeal
1 cup whole wheat pastry flour

Whole wheat biscuits – 14 biscuits.

1½ cups water
2 Tbsp coconut oil, melted
¼ tsp sea salt
2½ cups whole wheat flour or whole wheat pastry flour

Buckwheat and oatmeal biscuits – 14 biscuits.

1½ cups water
2 Tbsp coconut oil, melted
¼ tsp sea salt
½ cup rolled oats
1 cup buckwheat flour
1 cup whole wheat pastry flour

Comments – These simple recipes are low in fat and use no baking powder, soda, or yeast. Make different kinds of biscuits by using other flours such as rye or barley, or by adding nuts. The whole wheat biscuits can be made into cookies by using pastry flour and adding carob chips or cinnamon and raisins. See pages 16-17 on the use of oil.

Crisps

Procedure – Mix cold water and sea salt. Add flaked grain. Let stand until water is absorbed, 20 to 25 minutes. Spread thinly on an oiled baking sheet in 3-inch patties. Bake at 350 degrees for 30 to 40 minutes, or until crispy. See pages 16-17 on the use of oil

Oat crisp – Yield: 12 patties.

2 cups water
¼ tsp sea salt
3 cups rolled oats

Comments – Oat crisps are a light alternative to crackers. When mixing batter, it may seem too wet, yet the flakes will absorb most of the water. If there is liquid remaining, spoon some of the liquid onto each of the patties. For variety use rye or wheat flakes alone or in combination with rolled oats. Oat crisp can be made into a sweet cookie by adding nuts or currants or by replacing water with apple juice.

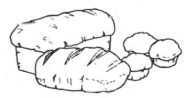

Pancakes and Waffles, Unleavened

Procedure – Mix water, sea salt, and grain, if used, separating lumps. Add flour. Lightly mix. Let stand 5 to 10 minutes. Batter should be pourable. For pancakes, ladle onto medium-hot, oiled skillet. Pan-fry the first side for 5 minutes or until pancake holds its shape, and the second side 2 to 3 minutes until browned. For waffles, ladle onto heated, well-oiled waffle iron. Bake until browned, 7 to 10 minutes.

Simple pancakes or waffles – 16 four-inch pancakes or 8 four-inch waffles.

> 2 cups water
> ⅛ tsp sea salt
> 2 cups whole-grain flour
> coconut oil for pan-frying

Pancakes or waffles with grain – 16 four-inch pancakes or 8 four-inch waffles.

> 2 cups water
> ⅛ tsp sea salt
> 1 cup cooled, cooked whole grain
> 2 cups whole-grain flour
> coconut oil for pan-frying

Comments – Pancakes with cooked grain are thicker than pancakes made with flour only, which are thin like crepes. Try using various grains and flours: cooked rice with whole wheat flour; cooked rice with buckwheat flour; cooked millet or cooked oatmeal with whole wheat flour. Also try roasting the flour, or adding currants, roasted seeds, or nuts. Top pancakes with maple syrup, thinned rice syrup, apple sauce, mashed cooked winter squash, Nut butter sauce, page 178 or Berry sauce, page 223. See pages 16-17 on the use of oil.

Batter Bread and Muffins, Leavened

Procedure – Preheat oven. Sift together dry ingredients. Whisk together wet ingredients. (If using egg, whisk egg and oil together first, then whisk with other wet ingredients.) Gently mix dry and wet ingredients. Add any nuts, raisins, or berries. Fold together. Fill oiled pan or muffin tins. Bake in preheated oven for time specified.

Cornbread – Use 8" x 10" pan. Bake at 450 degrees for 20 to 25 minutes.

2 cups corn flour
2 cups barley or whole wheat pastry flour
4 tsp baking powder
1 tsp sea salt
¼ cup coconut oil, melted
¼ cup maple syrup
2½ cups rice milk, soy milk, or water
add ¼ cup lightly toasted poppy seeds; add 1 egg and reduce liquid by ¼ cup; add ¼ tsp lemon extract, optional

Blueberry muffins – Bake at 400 degrees for 15 to 18 minutes. Paper liners can be used. In memory of Lil Myles. Yield: 24 muffins.

3 cups flour (whole wheat pastry, barley, unbleached white, or combination)
1 Tbsp baking powder
½ tsp sea salt
2 eggs
½ cup coconut oil, melted
¾ cup maple syrup or other sweetener
1 cup liquid, such as water, rice or soy milk, or juice
1 tsp vanilla extract
1 pint blueberries, 2 cups

Comments – Baking with baking powder produces light breads that can bake quickly. This recipe for corn bread is lighter than the unleavened recipe and is good for company and kids. The muffin recipe can be varied with different kinds of sweeteners, flours, liquids, and berries, fresh or frozen. Nuts can be added too. Cranberry muffins with walnuts and apple juice are delicious! See page 154 for comments on the use of eggs and pages 16-17 on the use of oil.

Dumplings

Procedure – Mix flour, baking powder if used, and sea salt. Mix boiling water with tahini, if used, then mix with flour. Knead in bowl for 1 minute. Form into ½-inch-diameter balls. Drop into boiling water or soup. Cover pot and simmer 5 minutes. Dumplings are done when they float.

Dumplings – 35 half-inch-diameter dumplings.

> 1 cup flour (whole wheat, whole wheat pastry, rice,
>   spelt, kamut, or buckwheat flour)
> pinch sea salt
> ½ cup boiling water

Dumplings with leavening – 35 half-inch-diameter dumplings.

> 1 cup flour (whole wheat, whole wheat pastry, rice,
>   spelt, kamut, or buckwheat flour)
> ½ tsp baking powder
> pinch sea salt
> 1 Tbsp tahini or almond butter
> ½ cup boiling water

Comments – Dumplings top soups nicely and are quick to make. To vary, roast the flour before mixing the batter.

Baking Mix

Procedure – Sift all ingredients together and store in a large tight container. Use within 2 weeks.

To make waffles: whisk all ingredients together. Ladle onto heated, well oiled waffle iron. Bake until browned, 7 to 10 minutes.

Basic baking mix – Yield: 3 cups

---

3 cups flour, any kind or a mixture, see comments
1 Tbsp baking powder
½ tsp sea salt
1 to 2 Tbsp arrowroot powder
⅛ tsp cinnamon

Waffles from baking mix – Yield: 6 four-inch waffles.

---

1 cup baking mix
1 egg, or 2 to 3 Tbsp water
1 cup water or rice milk

Comments – If you ever buy a baking mix, you may find it includes ingredients such as fillers or sweeteners you might not want, or even items detrimental to you or someone in your family. Here is a recipe you can adapt to create your own baking mix with the ingredients you want. Use for pancakes, waffles, muffins, quick breads, and cobblers. Vary it with the flours you like best, to introduce flours such as teff or garbanzo, and to add extra nutrition. Spices such as coriander and cinnamon can be added, too. Keep to the proportion of 1 teaspoon aluminum-free baking powder and ⅙ teaspoon sea salt per cup of flour.

Here are some combinations: 2 parts whole wheat pastry flour or barley flour, 1 part unbleached white flour, small amount of corn flour; 1 part whole wheat pastry flour or barley flour, 1 part buckwheat flour, 1 part rice flour; 2 parts whole wheat pastry flour or barley flour, 1 part teff, garbanzo, oat, or rice flour.

Desserts and Snacks

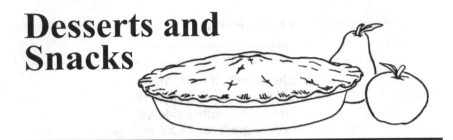

Use – Desserts enhance a meal. They add a finishing touch and can be elaborate or simple, exciting, entertaining, and/or relaxing depending on the ingredients used. This book includes desserts that can be made quickly, easily, and in small amounts. Many are cooked on top of the stove and use only one pan.

Desserts, especially those with sweeteners or fruits, are generally more yin and are used sparingly to several times a week depending on one's health and purpose. Many of the desserts in this chapter are appropriate for anyone wanting to avoid concentrated sweeteners, leavening agents, and excessive fats. Some desserts are made with vegetables and use no fruits or sweeteners.

Fruits – Wash fresh fruits before cutting. If fruit is not organic, you may wish to peel it. Juices and/or dried fruits can be used in place of sweeteners for lightly sweetened desserts.

Vegetables – Sweet potatoes, winter squash, and parsnips make delicious desserts. Use leftovers or simmer with sea salt up to 2 hours to increase their sweet flavor. Fill muffins or pies or use as an ingredient in puddings, breads, or cookies. Sweet potatoes can be served as a simple dessert by topping with roasted almonds or cashews.

Sea Salt – Sea salt brings out the natural sweetness of fruit. It also helps balance potassium in fruit and helps maintain acid/alkaline balance with grains. Use a high quality sea salt in your cooking.

Oil – Use good-quality oils in baking, see pages 16-17 for detailed information.

Baked Whole Fruit

Procedure – Mix stuffing ingredients, if used. Mixture should be moist and hold its shape. Stuff whole cored fruit or fruit cut in halves and cored. Place water and fruit, stuffed side up, in oiled baking dish. Cover dish. Bake at 350 degrees for 1 hour or until soft.

Baked apples – Yield: 6 to 12 pieces.

6 large apples, whole or halved, cored
Stuffing: optional
   2 Tbsp tahini
   2 to 3 tsp water or apple juice
   ½ tsp cinnamon
   ¼ tsp soy sauce
½ cup boiling water for baking dish

Baked pears – Yield: 6 to 12 pieces.

6 large pears, halved and cored
Stuffing: optional
   2 Tbsp tahini or almond butter
   2 to 3 tsp lemon juice
   ¼ tsp soy sauce
½ cup boiling water for baking dish

Comments – This procedure works best with firm fruits such as apples and pears because they hold their shape. Other fruits such as peaches and plums can be baked whole, but become soft and lose their shape.

Fruit Cobblers

Procedure – Fill oiled baking dish with fruit. Cover with grated rinds and sauce if used. Drizzle sweetener on top if used. For topping: sift dry ingredients together. Whisk wet ingredients together. Mix dry and wet ingredients together and fold with coconut or nuts if used. Spoon batter on top of fruit. Bake at 400 degrees for 40 to 45 minutes or 350 degrees for 1 hour or until fruit mixture is bubbly and cobbler is browned. See pages 16-17 on the use of oil.

Apple cobbler – 9″ x 9″ baking dish

4 cups apples, thinly sliced
¼ cup water or apple juice for baking dish
½ tsp grated lemon or orange rind
½ cup rice or maple syrup to drizzle on top, optional
Topping: 1 cup whole wheat pastry or barley flour
    1 tsp baking powder
    pinch sea salt
    pinch cinnamon
    1 Tbsp coconut oil, melted
    1 Tbsp maple syrup
    ½ cup rice milk or apple juice
    ¼ cup chopped walnuts, optional

Peach cobbler – 9″ x 9″ baking dish.

---

4 cups peaches, sliced
Sauce: ¼ cup apple juice
   ¼ tsp sea salt
   4 Tbsp arrowroot powder
   ¼ tsp grated lemon peel
   ¼ tsp coriander, optional
½ cup rice or maple syrup to drizzle on top, optional
Topping: 1 cup whole wheat pastry or barley flour
   1 tsp baking powder
   pinch sea salt
   pinch cinnamon
   1 Tbsp coconut oil, melted
   1 Tbsp maple syrup
   ½ cup rice milk or apple juice
   2 Tbsp shredded coconut, optional

Comments – Cobblers enhance seasonal fruit such as strawberries, plums, peaches, and blueberries singly or in combination. Many fruits bake well together. Try raspberries and peaches for instance. Arrange fruit in pan and drizzle rice or maple syrup on top to avoid bruising fruit and for extra flavor.

Make a sauce of juice, arrowroot powder, sea salt, and spices for fruits that are juicy. Use 1 tablespoon arrowroot powder per cup of fruit. Fruits become more juicy as they ripen so use more arrowroot for thickening ripe fruit. If you make your own Baking mix, page 213, it can be used in the topping. See additional notes under Fruit Crisps, page 218.

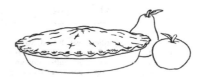

Fruit Crisps

Procedure – Fill oiled baking dish with fruit. Add water. Sprinkle cinnamon and sea salt on top of fruit. Make topping: mix flour, rolled oats, and sea salt; add oil and water; mix until moistened but still crumbly. Sprinkle topping on fruit. Cover dish (see comments). Bake at 400 degrees for 30 to 35 minutes or until fruit is soft. Remove cover and bake 15 minutes to crisp topping. See pages 16-17 on the use of oil.

Apple crisp – 9″ by 9″ baking dish

> 4 cups apples, thinly sliced
> ¼ cup water or apple juice
> ¼ tsp sea salt
> ½ tsp cinnamon
> Topping: ½ cup whole wheat pastry flour
>   1 cup rolled oats
>   ¼ tsp sea salt
>   2 Tbsp coconut oil, melted
>   3 Tbsp water, juice, or maple syrup

Comments – Crisps and cobblers are delicious and easy. Crisps are crunchy; cobblers are cake-like. Crisps and cobblers work well with almost any kind of fruit. Try pears, peaches, berries, or combinations. Cooked winter squash can be used, or cooked squash and raw apples together. For more sweetness, drizzle rice syrup on the cut fruit before sprinkling on topping. Vary topping by adding ¼ cup grated unsweetened coconut or chopped walnuts.

Cover or no cover? Cover fruit dishes for firm fruits such as apples and pears so the fruit bakes completely. Omit the cover for juicy fruits such as berries and stone fruits so excess liquid will steam off.

Sauce or no sauce? Juicy fruits such as berries and stone fruits release their own juice while baking. Make a sauce with arrowroot, see comments page 217, to thicken these juices. Firm fruits release less of their own juices. Add water or apple juice to the dish for baking.

Sautéed Fruit

Procedure – Heat oil in skillet. Add 1 layer of fruit. Brown for 1 to 2 minutes on each side. Add water and sea salt. Cover and bring to a boil. Steam over low heat for 10 minutes until water is evaporated.

Sautéed apples – Yield: 2 cups.

1 tsp light sesame oil or olive oil
2 large apples, thinly sliced, 3 cups
¼ cup water
pinch sea salt

Sautéed pears – Yield: 2 cups.

1 tsp light sesame oil or olive oil
2 large pears, thinly sliced, 3 cups
¼ cup water
pinch sea salt

Comments – This procedure works best with firm fruit such as apples and pears. It is good in the fall, and when you want a quick dessert or snack. Vary the recipes by adding a pinch of cinnamon, ginger, or nutmeg to the water and sea salt.

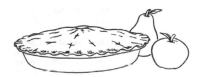

Stewed Dried Fruits

Procedure – Place dried fruit and water in pan. If dried fruit is hard, soak 15 to 20 minutes. Add sea salt after soaking. Cover and bring to a boil. Simmer over low heat for 20 to 30 minutes or until soft. Mash.

Stewed apricots – Yield: 2 cups.

> 1 cup dried apricots
> 1½ cups water
> ½ tsp sea salt

Stewed prunes – Remove prune pits, if needed, after cooking. Yield: 2 cups.

> 1½ cups prunes, whole or pitted
> 1½ cups water
> ½ tsp sea salt

Raisin sauce – Purée after cooking. Yield: 2 cups.

> 1½ cups raisins or currants
> 1½ cups water
> ½ tsp sea salt

Comments – Stewed dried fruits are often called compotes. Vary compotes with choice of dried fruits, singly or in combination, and seasonings. Ginger can be added as well as vanilla extract, cinnamon, coriander, or cardamom. Dried peach, raisin, ginger, cardamom, and sea salt is delicious. Fruit can be blended after cooking for a smoother texture. Serve separately, use as a topping for pancakes or biscuits, fill muffins, or add to cookies or puddings.

Fruit Sauces

Procedure – Place water or juice in pan. Add ingredients in order listed. Retain rice syrup and vanilla if used. Cover and bring to a boil. Simmer over low heat for the time indicated. Add rice syrup and vanilla extract at end of cooking. Purée in a blender or food processor for a smoother texture, or purée in a food mill to remove skins, if desired.

Applesauce – Simmer 30 minutes. Yield: 4 cups.

> 1 cup water or apple juice
> 3 pounds apples, cored and chopped, 8 cups
> 1 tsp sea salt

Peach sauce – Simmer 20 minutes. Yield: 4 cups.

> ½ cup water or apple juice
> 3 pounds peaches, pitted and chopped, 8 cups
> 1 tsp sea salt
> ¼ cup rice syrup

Cranberry sauce – Simmer 30 minutes. Yield: 5 cups.

> 1 cup water or apple juice
> ½ cup raisins
> 4 apples, cored and chopped, 4 cups
> 12 ounces cranberries, 3 cups
> 1 tsp sea salt
> 1 tsp vanilla extract

Comments – Classic fruit sauces require simple cooking. Many fruits from plums to apples to berries to combinations are suitable for cooking in this way. Sweeten with rice or maple syrup if fruit is tart. Vary sauces by adding cinnamon, cardamom, or lemon zest; or condense into a fruit butter through additional cooking. Simmer in an uncovered pan or slow cooker for 1 to 1½ hours until thick and deep-colored.

Fruit in Clear Sauce

Procedure – Bring water or juice, sea salt, and raisins, if used, to a boil. Simmer raisins 5 to 10 minutes over low heat until plump. Add fruit. Bring to a boil. Add dissolved arrowroot. Stir until thick and clear, 1 to 2 minutes. Remove from heat. Add flavoring.

Peaches in sauce – Yield: 3 cups.

1 cup water
¼ tsp sea salt
¼ cup raisins or currants
4 large peaches, pitted and cut into crescents, 4 cups
1 Tbsp arrowroot dissolved in 2 Tbsp water
Flavoring: ½ tsp vanilla or lemon extract

Blueberries and raspberries in sauce – Yield: 3½ cups.

1 cup apple juice
¼ tsp sea salt
1 cup blueberries
1 cup raspberries
2 Tbsp arrowroot dissolved in 3 Tbsp apple juice
Flavoring: ½ tsp vanilla or lemon extract

Comments – These recipes are used with stone fruits and berries, both of which lose their shape with cooking. The first uses raisins for sweetening; the second uses apple juice. Both are delicious served with Simple lemon cake, page 238, pancakes, waffles, couscous, or biscuits.

Substitute other stone fruits such as plums or apricots for the peaches, or other berries such as strawberries or boysenberries for blueberries. Fruits can also be mixed as desired.

Other Fruit Sauces

Raisin sauce to pour over fresh berries – Bring water, sea salt, and raisins to a boil. Simmer 5 to 10 minutes over low heat, until raisins are plump. Add dissolved arrowroot, and stir until thick and clear, 1 to 2 minutes. Cool 5 minutes. Pour over fruit. Yield: about ¾ cup sauce.

> 1 cup water
> ¼ tsp sea salt
> ½ cup raisins or currants
> 1 Tbsp arrowroot powder dissolved in 2 Tbsp cold water
> 2 to 3 cups fresh strawberries, blueberries, raspberries,
>   cherries, or cantaloupe

Berry sauce – Bring berries to a boil over low heat with sea salt. Simmer 5 to 10 minutes or until berries have released juice and mixture is bubbly. Add sweetener or apple sauce and thicken with dissolved arrowroot if needed. Yield: 2 cups.

> 1 pint strawberries, sliced, or blueberries, 2 cups
> ¼ tsp sea salt
> ¼ cup rice syrup or 1 cup applesauce
> 1 Tbsp arrowroot dissolved in 1 Tbsp water or juice,
>   optional

Comments – These two sauces are refreshing in the summer when fresh berries are available. Raisin sauce is good when wanting fresh fruit; berry sauce is good when wanting cooked berries. Both are delicious on waffles, pancakes, or simple cakes. For strawberry shortcake, make Berry sauce, using strawberries, and serve on Simple lemon cake, page 238.

Fruit and Grain Puddings

Procedure – Place all ingredients in pan, except flavoring and nuts, if used. Cover and bring to a boil. Simmer over low heat for the time indicated. Remove from heat. Stir in flavoring and/or nuts. Purée in blender or food processor for a smooth texture, if desired. Cool to set.

Apricot pudding – Simmer 30 minutes. For best results, purée in blender in small batches. Yield: 4½ cups.

4 cups water
¼ tsp sea salt
1 cup rolled oats
½ cup raisins
¼ cup dried apricots
Flavoring: ½ tsp vanilla extract

Rice pudding – Simmer 15 minutes. Yield: 6 cups.

3 cups soymilk
4 cups cooked brown rice
½ cup raisins
¼ tsp cinnamon
dash of vanilla extract
½ cup walnuts, roasted and chopped

Lemon pudding – Simmer 30 minutes. Yield: 5½ cups.

4 cups water
¼ tsp sea salt
1 cup millet, washed and drained
4 apples, cored and chopped, 4 cups
½ tsp grated lemon rind
Flavoring: 2 Tbsp lemon juice

Comments – These recipes feature grains that produce substantial puddings: rolled oats, cooked brown rice, and millet. My family enjoys their mild sweetness as puddings, but they can be served as a main course or for breakfast. They can be sweetened further if desired. Vary the recipes with choice of dried fruits, substituting juices for water, or by adding spices. Try: dried peach with rolled oats; rice pudding with dried ginger, cinnamon, cloves, and almonds; millet pudding cooked in strawberry and apple juice with raisins, almonds, and coriander, sweetened with maple syrup.

Soymilk Puddings

Procedure – Sprinkle sea salt and agar flakes over soy milk and bring to a boil over medium heat in an uncovered pan. Simmer 5 minutes or until flakes are dissolved. Mix tahini and maple syrup with diluted arrowroot and add to pan, stirring to mix. Remove from heat and add vanilla extract. Ladle into bowl and allow to set 1 to 1½ hours.

Vanilla pudding – Yield: 3½ cups.

¼ tsp sea salt
3 cups soymilk
3 Tbsp agar flakes
¼ cup tahini
¼ cup maple syrup
1 Tbsp arrowroot dissolved in ½ cup soymilk
1 tsp vanilla extract

Comments Soymilk is creamy and rich and when coupled with tahini, maple syrup, and agar flakes makes a wholesome pudding. Varieties of soymilk and tahini vary. If your pudding sets more thick than creamy, cut into squares and whip in blender. Vary this recipe by adding ¼ cup carob powder or by garnishing with roasted almonds.

Flour Puddings

Procedure – Heat oil in a pan. Add flour(s) and roast until fragrant, 1 to 2 minutes, stirring constantly with the back of a wooden spoon to smooth lumps. Remove from heat and cool 5 to 10 minutes. Whisk with 1 cup of cold liquid. Place over medium heat and add the rest of the cold liquid, stirring constantly. Add sea salt and spices if used. Cover and bring to a boil. Simmer over low heat for 30 minutes using a heat diffuser. Stir once or twice. Remove from heat. Add sweetener and flavoring if used. Cool to set.

Cornmeal pudding – Yield: 4 cups.

> 1 Tbsp light sesame oil or olive oil
> 1 cup fine cornmeal
> 4 cups apple juice
> ¼ tsp sea salt
> ½ tsp cinnamon

Carob pudding – Roast carob powder and flour together. Yield: 4 to 5 cups.

> 1 Tbsp light sesame oil or olive oil
> 4 Tbsp carob powder
> 1 cup barley or whole wheat pastry flour
> 4 to 5 cups water, or rice or soy milk
> ¼ tsp sea salt
> ¼ cup maple syrup
> Flavoring: 1 tsp vanilla extract

Comments – Flour puddings are cooked in a way similar to bechamel sauces, page 177. Vary with choice of flour, juice, and sweetener, and the addition of dried fruits and spices. Sweet rice flour with rice syrup, anise, and lemon extract is delicious.

Couscous Puddings

Procedure – Bring liquid to a boil. Add other ingredients. Cover and bring to a boil. Remove from heat. Let stand 10 minutes before serving or removing to a serving dish. Garnish when serving.

Couscous and blueberry pudding – Yield: 8 cups.

5 cups apple juice
¼ tsp sea salt
2 cups couscous
1 pint blueberries, 2 cups

Couscous and squash pudding – Yield: 4 cups.

2½ cups water
⅛ tsp sea salt
1 cup couscous
1 cup cooked mashed winter squash, such as butternut
Garnish: roasted almonds, pages 183-184

Comments – Couscous is a processed wheat product made from steamed (and then dried) semolina flour available in refined or whole wheat form. Couscous puddings cook quickly; use with ingredients such as berries or leftover cooked vegetables that also cook quickly. The couscous and squash pudding is designed for anyone avoiding concentrated sweeteners or fruit.

Vary these recipes by substituting sweet potatoes for the winter squash or strawberries for the blueberries. Rice syrup can be added for more sweetness if desired.

To make couscous cake, spoon pudding into a dampened pan, smooth top, and allow to set until cool. Serve with a fruit sauce on top. Couscous cooked in apple juice, with raisins, almonds, cinnamon, and vanilla extract makes a delicious cake.

Kanten Gelled Desserts

Procedure – Bring agar, liquid, and sea salt to a boil with lid ajar. Simmer over low heat until agar is dissolved, see comments. Add fruit other than berries, lemon rind, or sweetener next and bring to a boil. Dilute kuzu powder and add next; cook until clear, 1 to 2 minutes. Remove from heat. Cool in pan 5 to 10 minutes. Add flavoring and berries, if used. Ladle into serving dishes. Gel at room temperature for 1 to 1½ hours. If desired, refrigerate for faster jelling.

Peach and apple kanten – Yield: 6 cups.

1 Tbsp agar powder or 4 Tbsp agar flakes
4 cups apple juice, reserve 2 Tbsp to dissolve arrowroot
¼ tsp sea salt
4 medium peaches, sliced into crescents, 3 cups
1 Tbsp kuzu dissolved in 2 Tbsp apple juice
Flavoring: ½ tsp vanilla extract

Creamy lemon kanten – Yield: 4 cups.

1 Tbsp agar powder or 4 Tbsp agar flakes
3 cups water (or 2½ cups water, ½ cup rice milk)
¼ tsp sea salt
½ cup rice syrup
1 tsp grated lemon rind or lemon extract
2 Tbsp kuzu dissolved in 2 Tbsp water
Flavoring: ½ cup lemon juice, 1 large lemon

Orange kanten – Yield: 4 cups.

1 Tbsp agar powder or 4 Tbsp agar flakes
2 cups water
¼ tsp sea salt
¼ cup rice syrup
Flavoring: 2 cups orange juice

Strawberry kanten – Yield: 5½ cups

---

1 Tbsp agar powder or 4 Tbsp agar flakes
3¾ cups water
¼ tsp sea salt
1 pint strawberries, sliced , 2 cups
½ cup rice syrup
Flavoring: 6 Tbsp lime juice, 2 limes

Comments – Agar is a colorless and flavorless sea vegetable that is used to make kanten—a gelled dessert. Agar is high in minerals and is preferred over gelatin, which is a by-product of the cattle industry.

Agar commonly is available in three forms: bars, flakes, and powder. Each form is cooked for a different length of time until it dissolves and each gels a different quantity of liquid. The following proportions are general; check the package of the brand you are using.

Bars – Soak in liquid for 10 minutes; then cook 20 to 30 minutes to dissolve. A package of 2 bars will gel 5 cups liquid.

Flakes – Cook 5 to 10 minutes to dissolve. One tablespoon will gel 1 cup liquid.

Powder – Cook 2 to 3 minutes to dissolve. One tablespoon will gel 4 cups liquid.

This procedure is general and features juices and fruits. Use different juices and fruits such as apple juice with blueberries or apricot juice with cherries. Cook fruits such as plums, apricots, and peaches; pour cooked kanten over fruits such as berries, cherries, and grapes. Kuzu makes a creamy and soothing kanten; it complements fruit kantens well.

To set a kanten in shorter time, use more agar or less liquid, or pour cooked kanten over frozen fruit. Kanten can be gelled in a Rolled pie crust, pages 234-235, for a clear pie. Let cool slightly before pouring into a baked and cooled crust to gel.

Drop Cookies, Unleavened

Procedure – Cream oil or nut butter and sweetener together. Mix in liquid. Add sea salt, spices, extracts, dried fruit, and nuts. Add rolled oats and/or flours, mixing well. Place damp cloth over bowl. Let dough rest 10 to 15 minutes. Spoon onto an oiled baking sheet and flatten into 2-inch cookies, about ½-inch thick. Bake at 350 degrees for 20 to 30 minutes or until bottoms are browned. Cool on a rack.

Oatmeal and walnut cookies – Firm dough. Yield: 40 two-inch cookies.

¼ cup coconut oil, melted
2 cups water or apple juice
½ tsp sea salt
½ tsp cinnamon
½ cup raisins or currants
½ cup walnuts, chopped
2 cups rolled oats
3 cups whole wheat pastry flour

Sweet nut butter cookies – Firm dough. Try peanut butter with barley malt syrup, tahini with rice syrup, or almond butter with maple syrup. If sweeteners or butters are hard, heat with one-half of the liquid until softened; then mix with other ingredients. This recipe makes a mild, biscuit-like cookie. Yield: 40 two-inch (or 30, 2½-inch) cookies.

½ cup nut or seed butter
¼ cup sweetener
1 cup water
½ tsp sea salt
¼ tsp vanilla extract
3 cups whole wheat pastry flour

Applesauce and oatmeal cookies – Soft dough. Yield: 20 two-inch cookies.

2 Tbsp coconut oil, melted
1 cup applesauce (sweetener)
1 cup water
¼ tsp sea salt
½ tsp cinnamon
2 cups rolled oats
1 cup whole wheat pastry flour

Squash and almond cookies – Soft dough. Drop cookies onto sheet, and place one almond on top of each before baking. Yield: 24 two-inch cookies.

2 Tbsp coconut oil, melted
2 cups cooked winter squash, mashed (sweetener)
1 cup water
¼ tsp sea salt
2 tsp fresh ginger juice, optional
½ tsp cinnamon
2½ cups brown rice or whole wheat pastry flour
almonds

Comments – These recipes are designed for anyone avoiding baking powder. The squash cookies are appropriate for anyone also avoiding concentrated sweeteners or fruit. Baking times are longer than for cookies that have baking powder. Make cookies 2 to 2½ inches in diameter as larger sizes do not bake as well.

The dough for these cookies can be firm or soft. Soft doughs have more liquid, but should hold their shape when placed on the baking sheet. Firm doughs have more flour but should be pliable and not too stiff when placed on the baking sheet. Vary these recipes with different fruit or nut butters, as well as nuts, sweeteners, spices, and dried fruit. For people with wheat allergy, substitute barley, oat, or rice flour. Drop cookies can also be made from the batters for Biscuits, unleavened, page 208, or Crisps, page 209. See pages 16-17 on the use of oil.

Drop Cookies, Leavened

Procedure – Sift flour with baking powder, sea salt, and spices. Cream oil with sweetener. Add any other liquid or flavorings. Mix in flour mixture, then any rolled oats, raisins, chips, or nuts. Spoon onto oiled baking sheet and flatten into 2-inch cookies, ½-inch thick. Bake 350 degrees for 12 to 14 minutes until browned. See pages 16-17 on the use of oil.

Carob chip cookies – Yield: about 12 two-inch cookies.

1 cup barley or whole wheat pastry flour
1 tsp baking powder
pinch of sea salt
¼ cup coconut oil, melted
¼ cup maple syrup
1 tsp vanilla extract
¼ cup good-quality (non-hydrogenated) carob chips

Oatmeal Raisin Cookies – Yield: 24, 2½-inch cookies.

2 cups flour: whole wheat pastry, barley, oat, or combination
1 Tbsp baking powder
¼ tsp sea salt
½ cup coconut oil, melted
½ cup maple syrup
1 tsp vanilla extract
1 cup rolled oats
½ cup raisins
½ cup chopped walnuts

Comments – Kids and guests love cookies. These recipes bake more quickly than the unleavened recipes. Vary by substituting good-quality chocolate chips for carob chips or dates and almonds for raisins and walnuts. Use aluminum-free baking powder.

Pressed Pie Crust

Procedure – For pressed pie crust: Mix flour and sea salt. Rub in oil by hand. Mix in rolled oats. Sprinkle a small amount of water over the dough with the fingers and mix with a fork. Sprinkle more water and gently mix until dough holds together. Add only enough water so dough sticks together and is still springy. Lightly mix. Avoid kneading as the crust can become tough. Press into an oiled pie tin. See pages 16-17 on the use of oil.

For flourless pie crust: In a food processor, process walnuts, rolled oats, coconut, if used, and sea salt until crumbly. Add other ingredients and process until moistened. Press into an oiled pie tin.

Fill and bake as per filling recipes, pages 236-237. If using with a gelled filling, bake at 350 degrees for 15 to 20 minutes.

Pressed pie crust – 1 crust for 9-inch pie.

---

2 cups whole wheat pastry flour
¼ tsp sea salt
¼ cup coconut oil, melted
½ cup rolled oats
6 to 7 Tbsp cold water

Pressed pie crust, flourless – 1 crust for 9-inch pie.

---

1 cup walnuts
2 cups rolled oats
¼ cup shredded coconut, optional
¼ tsp sea salt
2 Tbsp coconut oil, melted
2 Tbsp maple syrup or rice milk
½ cup water

Comments – Pressed pie crusts are thicker than rolled pie crusts. They complement vegetable fillings well and can be made without sweetening if desired. Vary the pressed pie crust recipe by using part sweet brown rice flour or brown rice flour. Use ¼ cup rice flour to 1¾ cups whole wheat pastry flour. Another variation is to add shredded, unsweetened coconut or chopped nuts. Vary the flourless recipe by substituting almonds for walnuts. Process in food processor first before processing with rolled oats and sea salt.

Rolled Pie Crust

Procedure – Mix flour and sea salt. Rub oil in by hand, smoothing lumps. (See illustration.) Sprinkle a small amount of water over dough with the fingers and mix with a fork. Sprinkle and add more water until dough holds together. Add only enough water so dough sticks together and is still springy. Lightly mix. Avoid kneading as the crust can become tough.

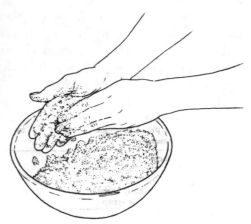

Separate into 2 parts. Roll the first part on a lightly floured surface such as waxed or parchment paper or a counter top, dusting dough with flour so rolling pin doesn't stick. Roll to 12-inch diameter, ¼-inch thick. Place in an oiled pie tin. Trim any dough extending over the edge of the pie tin with a table knife. If needed, bake bottom crust at 350 degrees for 10 minutes, see comments.

Fill with pie filling. For pie with top crust, roll out second part. Place on top of filling and trim extending dough. Slit top crust to allow steam to escape. If making a lattice top, cut dough into strips and lay strips crosswise on top of filling. Moisten around the edges between the top and bottom crust. Seal edges together by pinching between the thumb and forefinger. Bake as per filling recipes, pages 236-237. For a one-crust pie, halve the recipe.

Rolled pie crust – 2 crusts for 9-inch pie.

---

3 cups flour such as whole wheat pastry, barley, white,
    or mixture
¼ tsp sea salt
½ cup coconut oil, melted
about ½ cup cold water

Comments – This is perhaps the most difficult dessert recipe in this book as using whole grain flour to make a light and flaky pie crust takes thought and care. Whole wheat pastry flour becomes glutinous easily so work gently and quickly. Vary this basic crust with choice of flour. Barley, brown rice, or sweet rice flours are more delicate than whole wheat pastry and can be used in combination, such as ½ cup rice flour and 2½ cups pastry flour. White flour can be used half and half or 2 cups whole wheat pastry and 1 cup white flour.

Coconut oil bakes well and produces a tender crust, especially when combined with white flour. See pages 16-17 on the use of oil.

If the dough tears while rolling or placing into pie pan, patch it rather than kneading together and rolling out again. Avoid overworking the dough. Trimmings can be sprinkled with cinnamon and baked as cookies.

Bake the bottom crust before filling with berries or other fillings that contain more moisture, so crust won't become soggy. Prick holes in crust so air can escape and bake at 350 degrees for 10 minutes. In addition, use a lattice top crust to allow excess moisture to steam off while baking. If dough will be used for a gelled filling, prick holes in it and bake at 350 degrees for about 15 minutes or until browned. Cool, then fill.

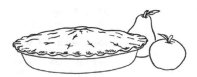

Pie Fillings

Procedure – Mix all ingredients in the order listed, adding one kind at a time. Fill pie crust. Cover with top crust if specified; crimp edges together and slit top crust. Bake at 350 degrees for the time indicated.

Squash pie – 9-inch pie. Use flourless pressed pie crust. Purée ingredients in food processor and thin to the consistency of thick apple sauce. Bake 1 hour or until filling has set.

3½ cups cooked Winter squash, page 99
¼ to ½ cups water from cooking squash
1 egg, optional
¼ cup maple syrup, optional
½ tsp cinnamon
¼ tsp nutmeg
¼ tsp cloves

Squash and apple pie – 9-inch pie. Use rolled pie crust with top crust. Bake 1 hour.

1 Tbsp whole wheat pastry or barley flour
½ tsp cinnamon
⅛ tsp sea salt
½ tsp grated lemon rind
¼ cup raisins or currants
2 cups apples, thinly sliced
2 cups cooked Winter squash, mashed, page 99

Sweet potato pie – 9-inch pie. Use pressed pie crust. Fill, garnish with pecans, and bake 45 to 55 minutes.

3 cups cooked Sweet potatoes, mashed, page 98
1 to ½ cups water
½ tsp cinnamon
Garnish: pecans

Apple or peach pie – 9-inch pie. Use rolled pie crust with top crust for apple pie and lattice top for peach pie. Mix all ingredients but sweetener. Fill crust and drizzle sweetener on top. Cover with top crust or lattice. Bake 1 hour or until crust is browned and filling is bubbly.

---

2 to 4 Tbsp whole wheat pastry or barley flour, see comments
½ tsp cinnamon
¼ tsp sea salt
½ tsp grated lemon rind
4 cups apples or peaches, thinly sliced
½ cup rice syrup or maple syrup for peach pie, optional for apple pie

---

Comments – A 9-inch pie needs 4 cups of filling, which can be fruit, vegetable, or a combination of fruit and vegetable.

Make fruit pies with apples, peaches, strawberries, cherries, or other fruit, singly or in combination. Use a rolled pie crust with a top crust, either solid or lattice. Thicken the juices with flour and increase the quantity of flour for fruit such as peaches and berries that release a lot of juice. Mix flour with sea salt and spices in order to distribute the spices evenly. To avoid bruising fruit, drizzle sweetener on top of fruit.

Make vegetable pies from winter squash, sweet potatoes, or parsnips, singly or in combination. Mash or purée cooked vegetables with other ingredients until soft but not runny. Filling will set while baking. Use a pressed or rolled pie crust without a top crust. Leftover cooked vegetables bake well but allow more time if vegetables are cold.

For vegetable and fruit pies, mix fruit with the flour mixture and then with the cooked mashed vegetables. Try other combinations such as pear and squash, or apple and parsnip. Add raisins or drizzle sweetener on top. Use a rolled pie crust with or without a top crust.

For gelled pies, bake any pie crust completely and cool. Make kanten dessert per recipe on pages 228-229. Pour into shell when kanten has cooled but has not set. Refrigerate to set. Try Creamy lemon kanten, page 228, in Rolled pie crust, page 235.

Cakes

Procedure – Preheat oven. Sift flour(s) with baking powder, sea salt, and spices. Mix liquid ingredients; if using egg, mix with oil before adding sweetener, or other liquids. Gently mix flour mixture into wet mixture. Pour into oiled baking pan and bake as directed. See pages 16-17 on the use of oil.

For glaze: Boil rice syrup with water and sea salt for 2 to 3 minutes. Add diluted arrowroot and stir until thickened. Remove from heat and add lemon juice. Pour on top of cooled cake.

For frosting: Bring maple syrup, water, and sea salt to a boil. Remove from heat, add vanilla extract and carob chips, stirring to melt the chips. Add peanut butter. Spread frosting on cooled cake.

Simple lemon cake with glaze – Use a 9″ x 13″ baking pan. Bake at 350 degrees for 30 to 35 minutes. Glaze yield: 1 cup.

3 cups flour: whole wheat pastry, barley, or combination
1 Tbsp baking powder
½ tsp sea salt
1 egg, optional, or ¼ cup water
½ cup coconut oil, melted
½ cup maple syrup
1 tsp lemon extract
¾ cup rice milk, soy milk, or water
Glaze: ¼ cup rice syrup
   ¼ cup water
   pinch of sea salt
   1 Tbsp arrowroot diluted in ¼ cup water
   ¼ cup lemon juice

Carob cake with frosting – Use a 9″ x 13″ baking pan. Bake at 350 degrees for 30 to 35 minutes. Frosting yield: 1½ cups.

---

1 cup carob flour
3 cups flour: whole wheat pastry, barley, white, or combination
1 Tbsp baking powder
½ tsp sea salt
1 egg, optional, or ¼ cup water
½ cup coconut oil, melted
1 tsp vanilla extract
½ cup maple syrup
1 cup applesauce
1½ cups apple juice
Frosting: ¼ cup maple syrup
   ¼ cup water
   pinch of sea salt
   ½ tsp vanilla extract
   1 cup good-quality (non-hydrogenated) carob chips
   ¼ cup peanut butter

Comments – These recipes are current favorites in my house as they are simple and quick, especially when using the Baking mix, page 213. They also lend themselves well to inspiration and variety.

Vary the Simple lemon cake by substituting vanilla extract for lemon extract. Serve with Berry sauce, page 223, using strawberries, for strawberry shortcake. Make spice cake by adding cinnamon, cloves, nutmeg, coriander, and walnuts. Serve with applesauce. Vary the glaze by substituting orange juice for lemon juice. Orange juice can be increased to ½ cup and the water decreased accordingly.

The Carob cake with frosting makes a festive, brownie-type birthday cake. Vary by substituting chocolate chips for the carob chips, or by adding carob chips, chocolate chips, or walnuts to the cake batter. Vary the frosting by substituting almond butter for peanut butter. For either cake, substitute flours, such as rice flour or oat flour, in the proportion of ½ cup rice or oat flour to 2½ cups barley or whole wheat pastry flour so the cake won't be too crumbly.

Granola

Procedure – Mix oil, sweetener, and sea salt. Heat if needed to make the mixture workable. Add remaining ingredients, except dried fruit, in the order listed, one kind at a time. Mix well after each addition.

Spread 4 cups on a 11″ by 17″ baking sheet in a layer ½-inch thick. Bake at 350 degrees for 20 to 25 minutes until browned and crisp. Stir every 7 to 10 minutes. Remove from baking sheet to bowl and add dried fruit. Cool, then store.

Granola – Yield: 8 cups.

¼ cup coconut oil, melted, see pages 16-17
½ cup rice syrup, barley malt, or maple syrup
½ tsp sea salt
½ cup sunflower seeds
1 cup almonds, chopped
6 cups rolled oats
1 cup currants or raisins

Comments – Granola varies easily; there are infinite possibilities of nuts, flakes, and dried fruits. Follow the simple guideline of: mixing oil, sweetener, and sea salt; and then adding other ingredients one kind at a time with those of smallest measure first. Add fruit after baking. Try these ingredients: cinnamon, vanilla extract, coconut flakes, pumpkin seeds, hazel nuts, wheat or rye flakes, dried apricots, dried prunes, and dried apples.

Granola can be unsweetened, too. Use ½ cup water instead of the ½ cup sweetener, and follow basic procedure. Serve granola with water, Grain milk, page 246, or soymilk.

Popcorn

Procedure – Heat pan over medium heat. Add oil, popping corn, and sea salt. Cover. For a small stainless steel pan, shake pan every 5 to 10 seconds. For a larger pan or wok, use chopsticks as needed to stir popcorn. As corn starts to pop consistently, shake continually until all corn is popped, about 7 to 10 minutes.

Popcorn – Fills a 2-quart pan.

1 to 4 Tbsp coconut oil, melted
½ cup popping corn
pinch sea salt

Comments – Popcorn pops quickly when the pan and oil are hot. For the first batch, heat the pan for 15 seconds. A second batch will pop in less time than the first batch, because the pan is already hot. In addition, less oil is needed for a second batch.

Use a lightweight stainless steel pan or wok. A wok works well as the heat is concentrated at the bottom of the pan, reducing the chance of burning.

Sea salt brings out flavor, but too much will hinder popping. The sea salt cooks into the corn so less is needed afterwards. If desired, sprinkle or spray soy sauce on hot popcorn (use clean spray bottle); or roast seeds, sprinkle them with soy sauce, and mix with popcorn.

Popping corn stored in the refrigerator pops better as it retains moisture.

Trail Mixes

Procedure – Roast seeds or nuts individually, pages 183-184. While still hot, sprinkle with a small amount of soy sauce. Let cool, then mix all ingredients.

Simple trail mix – Yield: 2 cups.

1 cup sunflower seeds
½ cup almonds
soy sauce, small amount
½ cup raisins or currants

Trail mix with puffed cereal – Yield: 20 cups.

1½ cups almonds
1½ cups walnuts
1½ cups peanuts
1½ cups sunflower seeds
1½ cups dried apples
1½ cups raisins
1½ cups pitted prunes
10 cups puffed rice, 1 bag

Comments – Trail mixes are easy to make and can be made in quantity to last for traveling or camping. Roast the seeds to make more digestible and add soy sauce for balance and flavor. Vary the recipe or proportions with choice of seeds, nuts, dried fruits, and puffed cereal grains. Try shredded or flaked coconut; dried apricots, blueberries, or cherries; carob chips after nuts or seeds are completely cooled; or anything else that suits your fancy.

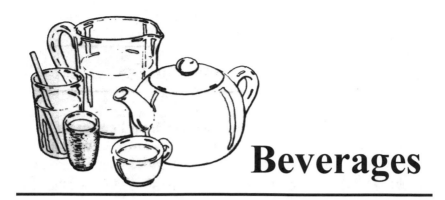

Beverages

Use – Many delicious beverages are used to complement a whole foods diet, from simple tea that ends a meal to thicker substantial drinks that enhance a meal.

Water – Water is the necessary ingredient in beverages. Choose a pure water to prepare teas and for daily drinking. Spring or filtered water is preferred over tap or distilled.

Consumption – Prepare beverages fresh and serve at a comfortable temperature. Avoid icy drinks or consuming large quantities of beverages with meals as they can inhibit digestion. For specific medicinal teas and beverages seek a qualified health-care practitioner or consult the index for recommended books.

Bancha Twig Tea

Procedure – Add tea to cold water. Cover pan or teapot and bring to a boil. For strong tea, simmer 15 to 20 minutes, then serve. For mild tea, simmer 3 to 5 minutes, then steep 15 to 20 minutes before serving.

Bancha twig tea – Yield: 4 cups.

> 1 Tbsp bancha twig tea
> 4 cups cold water

Comments – Bancha twig tea (or kukicha) is made from the roasted lower leaves and twigs of the tea bush. Like all tea, it contains some caffeine. However, the lower leaves and twigs contain less than outer leaves, and the leaves and twigs are roasted, which further reduce the effect of the caffeine. Bancha twig tea is a soothing tea which can be served every day.

Use a glass or enameled teapot to simmer and steep tea. The twig tea can be used for more than one pot of tea. With each new pot, add 1 tablespoon new twigs for 4 to 5 cups cold water. Discard when twigs accumulate to a ½-inch layer.

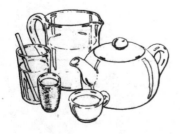

Grain Coffee and Tea

Procedure – To prepare grain, wash and drain 1 cup whole or pearled barley, whole wheat, brown rice, or a combination. Place in a dry skillet (no oil). Roast over medium to low heat until grain has popped, is very fragrant, and is turning dark brown, almost black. Stir often; after 30 minutes, stir continuously. It will take from 45 to 60 minutes to roast completely. For grain coffee, grind the hot roasted grain in a blender or a hand grain mill until it is powder. Cool. Store in a glass jar. For grain tea, do not grind. Cool roasted grain and store in a glass jar.

To make coffee or tea, add cooled, prepared grain to cold water. Bring to a boil. Simmer 15 to 20 minutes. Steep 10 minutes before serving. For grain tea, strain when serving.

Grain coffee – Yield: 5 cups.

2 Tbsp grain powder
5 cups cold water

Grain tea – Yield: 5 cups.

2 Tbsp prepared whole grain
5 cups cold water

Comment – Grain tea is clear and light in color. Grain coffee is thicker and darker in color than grain tea. Both are available ready made, but are fresher when homemade.

Take care to roast completely and uniformly as properly roasted grain can keep over a year. Grain can be used a second time for tea. Add 1 tablespoon more roasted grain for 5 cups water. After making tea, the whole grain can be cooked until soft for use as a porridge.

When purchasing grain coffee or tea, choose products that are free of dyes or commercial sweeteners. Use in the same proportion as listed above or follow directions on the package.

Grain Milk

Procedure – Cook rice by boiling for 1 hour, page 58, or pressure cooking for 45 minutes, page 68. Cook rolled oats by simmering 30 minutes, page 60. Strain for use as milk. Reserve grain and use in Fruit and Grain Puddings, page 224, or other use.

Grain milk – Yield: 5½ cups.

> 1 cup brown rice, rolled oats, or kokkoh mixture; wash
>   and soak rice before cooking
> pinch of sea salt
> 8 cups water

Kokkoh – Roast separately, page 62. Cool and mix together. Yield: 2½ cups.

> 1 cup brown rice, roasted
> ½ cup sweet brown rice, roasted
> ½ cup whole oats, roasted
> 1 Tbsp sesame seeds, roasted
> 2 Tbsp azuki beans, roasted

Comments – Kokkoh is macrobiotic grain milk recommended by George Ohsawa as appropriate food for a baby. Strain to make milk or grind in a baby-food grinder for the whole food. It can be sweetened with rice syrup if desired. Kokkoh is included here as an example of grain milk, not as a formula substitute or as a main food source for a newborn. I fed my babies kokkoh as supplemental food, sometimes making it thick as cream and other times thin as milk. When my children were young and when this book was first published, packaged soy and/or rice milks were not available.

Serve grain milk hot or at room temperature, over granola or puffed cereals, or as an ingredient in puddings or soups. Brown rice or rolled oat grain milk can be cooked and sweetened with raisins.

Umeboshi Kuzu Drink

Procedure – To make ginger juice, grate fresh ginger root on a fine grater. Japanese graters are handy because they have a small liquid reservoir. Squeeze out the juice. Place all ingredients in pan and heat over low to medium heat, stirring often. The mixture will turn from opaque to clear. Bring to a boil and remove from heat.

Umeboshi kuzu drink – Yield: 1 cup.

1 cup water or cool bancha twig tea
1 medium umeboshi, whole or broken into several
    pieces, including pit
1 tsp to 1 Tbsp kuzu powder
few drops to ¼ tsp ginger juice, freshly squeezed
few drops to ¼ tsp soy sauce

Comments – Umeboshi kuzu drink is a macrobiotic drink reported to be useful for many ailments from headaches to diarrhea to hangovers! I usually use this drink as a pick-me-up or when someone in my family has had a cold or flu. It is mild in flavor and is soothing for the digestive tract. Vary with the quantity of kuzu for a thicker drink. Vary the amount of ginger juice and soy sauce for flavor.

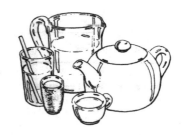

Mulled Juices

Procedure – Place all ingredients in a pan. Cover. Bring to a boil. Simmer 15 minutes over low heat. Strain whole spices when serving.

Small amount – Yield: 2½ to 3 cups.

2 cups apple juice or apple juice blend
½ to 1 cup water
pinch sea salt
pinch ground cinnamon

Large amount – Yield: 20 cups.

1 gallon apple juice
1 quart water
½ tsp sea salt
4 cinnamon sticks
¼ tsp whole cloves

Comments – Mulled juices, also known as mulled ciders, are festive and warming for holidays and during cool temperatures. Traditional recipes call for apple juice with sea salt and cinnamon to make a sweet blend. Add other juices such as strawberry, apricot, peach, orange, or lemon to apple for variety. Mulled apple cider can be varied by simmering with nutmeg, allspice, organic orange or lemon peel, or a vanilla bean.

Sparkling Juices

Procedure – Mix juices if using more than one kind. Add mineral water just before serving.

Grape Soda – Yield 1½ cups.

1 cup grape juice
½ cup carbonated mineral water

Fruit Punch – Yield: 36 cups.

1 gallon apple juice
1 quart grape juice
1 quart apple and strawberry juice
3 quarts carbonated mineral water, lemon, lime, or plain

Comments – Sparkling juice refreshes in the summer. Carbonated mineral water loses its fizz after 20 minutes; add just before serving. Serve at room temperature or slightly chilled. Use any juice or combination as desired: grape, apple, pear, apricot, or berry with apple, in a proportion of 2 parts juice to 1 part carbonated mineral water.

If preferred, use herbal tea in place of mineral water. Brew 1 tea bag per cup of water and double the amount of juice. For example, mix 1 cup of brewed raspberry or other berry tea to 2 cups apple juice.

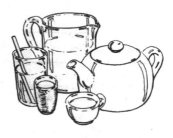

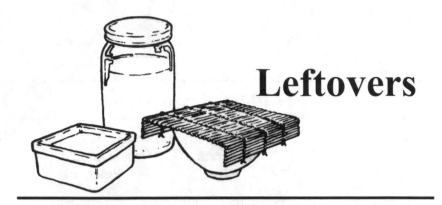

Leftovers

Use – The word "leftover" implies food that is merely reheated and served. But foods that are left over can be mixed together to form new dishes and meals. Sometimes, it is practical to cook extra so there will be intentional leftovers. Some dishes are time consuming to make; if some ingredients are already cooked, preparation is simplified. For example, leftover cooked winter squash can be used as a filling for pie or muffins; medley salads or casseroles become easy when the grain or noodles are already cooked.

Ease of mixing – The more simple the leftover, the more versatile. Plain rice combines with more dishes than rice cooked with vegetables. A dish seasoned only with oil, sea salt, or soy sauce is easier to incorporate into a new dish than a dish with many seasonings.

Reheating leftovers – If leftovers have been refrigerated, reheat for better flavor. When food will be served in the same way, reheat by placing ½ to 1 inch of water in bottom of pan, laying leftovers on top, heating to boiling, simmering 3 to 4 minutes, then mixing. Rice and other grains heat through well without burning. A second way to heat leftovers is to place 1 inch of water in the bottom of a large pot. Place the whole Pyrex or stainless steel bowl of leftovers into the pot. Cover. Steam 10 minutes. This method avoids adding extra water to the dish. A third way is to place a plate of food in a bamboo steamer and steam to reheat.

Balance – For optimal balance and appeal when serving leftovers, add something fresh to the meal such as a garnish, roasted seeds, a freshly cooked vegetable side dish, or a salad.

Burgers

Procedure – Combine all ingredients, except oil, and mix well. Mixture should be firm. Heat oil, see pages 16-17, in a skillet. Spoon mixture onto skillet. Flatten into burger shapes. Cover and fry 7 minutes. Uncover, and fry other side 5 minutes. Add more oil to skillet for second batch.

Grain burgers – Mix grain and water first to separate clumps of grain. Yield: 8 three-inch patties.

1 cup cooked rice, millet, or buckwheat
1 cup water
1 Tbsp barley miso
½ small onion, finely minced, optional, ½ cup
1 cup whole wheat pastry flour
1 Tbsp coconut oil for skillet, or more

Salmon burgers – Yield: 8 three-inch patties.

½ cup cooked salmon, bones removed and mashed
1 small onion, finely minced, 1 cup
2 cloves garlic, pressed
¼ tsp dried mustard powder
1 tsp ginger juice
2 tsp soy sauce
1 egg or ¼ cup water
¾ cup whole wheat pastry flour
1 Tbsp coconut oil for skillet, or more

Comments – Burgers are a perfect way to utilize leftovers and can be made using any leftover grain, fish, flour, or leftover noodle cooking water. Endless variations are possible. Add mashed tofu or finely chopped walnuts or sunflower seeds; fold in finely minced carrots, parsley, celery, mushrooms, or scallions; season with powdered garlic, oregano, or mustard; fry with more oil. Cover the skillet to cook the minced vegetables thoroughly as well as to contain spatters. Have fun!

Fried Grain Slices

Procedure – While it is still hot, scoop cooked polenta, millet, or teff into a loaf pan. Smooth the top of the loaf. Let stand until firm and completely cool. When ready to fry, turn the loaf out of the pan and slice into ½-inch thick pieces. Heat oil in skillet. Pan-fry, uncovered, until browned, 3 to 5 minutes each side.

Fried grain slices

cooked and cooled polenta, millet, or teff
1 Tbsp coconut oil for skillet

Comments – Fried grains slices can be made from polenta, millet, or teff that has been boiled, sautéed and boiled, roasted and boiled, sautéed and boiled with vegetables, pages 59-65, or pressure cooked, page 69. Herbs and spices embrace polenta and millet and can be used liberally to create main courses or desserts as desired.

Serve plain, with soy sauce, with maple syrup or a fruit sauce for dessert, or with beans and vegetables for a main course.

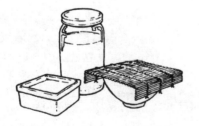

Grain and Vegetable Casseroles

Procedure – Mix ingredients together, adding extra water or liquid if needed. Mixture should be moist yet hold its shape when placed into the baking pan. Place in an oiled pan. Cover, if desired, to prevent drying out. Bake 30 minutes at 350 degrees.

Casserole combination ideas

Cooked noodles, cooked tofu sauce, and fresh chopped scallions

---

Cooked rice, layered vegetables, and cooked nut butter sauce

Cooked polenta, cooked beans, and fresh chopped scallions

Cooked noodles, cooked bechamel sauce, cooked fish, and fresh chopped scallions

---

Comments – Most casseroles are made of precooked foods and a sauce. Leftovers are ideal ingredients in casseroles and can be mixed in any desired proportions. Generally, use grains, vegetables, and a sauce or water. Casseroles can be made by layering leftovers into the pan rather than mixing. For example, place noodles in pan, top with steamed vegetables, and ladle bechamel sauce over all.

Ideally, use some fresh ingredients along with leftover ingredients when making casseroles. If all ingredients are leftover, include seasoning or scallions to add freshness. Another way is to cook some new ingredients for use in the casserole dish. For example, to make tamale pie: cook polenta, gently press into pie tin, spoon leftover beans into polenta "shell" and add caramelized onions on top, either leftover or freshly made. Bake at 350 degrees for 30 minutes. Freshly cooked millet can be used as a shell also, topping with beans, cooked squash, or sweet potatoes; or steamed vegetables and bechamel sauce.

Grain and Vegetable Pies

Procedure – Make Rolled pie crust, page 234. Place bottom crust in pie tin. Mix filling. It should be moist and soft, yet not runny. Place filling into bottom crust. Place top crust on top of filling, if desired. Crimp bottom and top crust together and slit top crust to allow steam to escape. Bake 25 to 30 minutes at 350 degrees.

Grain and vegetable pie combination ideas

Cooked rice, cooked hijiki, water, and fresh chopped scallions

Cooked green vegetables, cooked polenta or millet, and fresh-beaten egg

Cooked vegetables, cooked fish, and cooked bechamel sauce

Cooked vegetables, cooked beans, and soy sauce

Comments – Pie fillings should be moist; they will set as they bake. Since there is a crust, use a higher proportion of vegetables to grain; or make a vegetable-only pie, mixing with beaten egg if desired. For a 9-inch pie, use 4 cups of filling; 3 parts vegetables to 1 part grain.

Just as with casseroles, pies can be made with some ingredients leftover and some freshly cooked. Try a tofu vegetable pie with leftover cooked vegetables; mash tofu and mix with soy sauce, tahini, and garlic or other herbs; moisten with soymilk.

Grain and Vegetable Porridges

Procedure – Place ingredients in a pot with water, soup, or liquid at bottom; firm or solid ingredients at top. Use at least the same amount of cooked grain as liquid. Cover and bring to a boil. Simmer 15 minutes over low heat. Add soy sauce or miso to taste.

Grain and vegetable porridge ideas

Leftover miso soup, cooked rice, and fresh minced scallions

Leftover vegetable soup, cooked rice, and hard bread crusts

Water, cooked vegetables, and cooked noodles

Water, cooked vegetables, cooked beans, and cooked grain

Leftover vegetable soup, cooked noodles, and cooked fish

Comments – Commonly called "ojiya" in Japanese, these thick, seasoned porridges can be made with almost any leftovers. If leftover vegetables or noodles are larger than bite-sized, cut into smaller sizes before making into porridge. For freshness, add fresh ginger juice to the seasoning or garnish with roasted seeds or scallions.

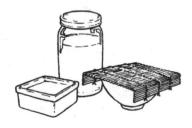

Ideas for Using Leftovers

Grains

Serve with roasted nuts, seeds, or a sauce.

Add to soup to heat through.

Mix with cooked vegetables. Cook vegetables by layering, page 83, or by simmering, page 97. During the last 5 minutes of cooking, lay grain on top of vegetables to heat through.

Fry with vegetables. Sauté or stir-fry vegetables, page 88. Add grain during last 5 minutes of cooking to heat through. Season.

Cook leftover grain into a new grain dish. Cook bulgur, polenta, or oatmeal with the usual amount of water, adding leftover cooked rice for the full cooking time.

Make into grain milk, page 246; casserole, pie, or porridge, pages 253-255; pancakes, page 210; pudding, page 224; salad, page 171; or bread, page 204 or 206.

Noodles

Serve with sauce or garnish.

Add to soup and heat through.

Make into salad, page 171; sea vegetable dish, page 127; casserole, page 253; or porridge, page 255.

Vegetables

Heat with cooked grain. Garnish with roasted seeds.

Add to soup.

Make into casserole, pie, or porridge, pages 253-255; bread, page 205; or muffins, page 207.

Make into a dessert or topping, especially if winter squash, sweet potatoes, or parsnips. See pages 227, 231, and 236.

Soups

> Serve over grains, noodles, or muffins.
>
> Heat with cooked grains or noodles.
>
> Thin soup and cook noodles or dumplings in it.
>
> Make porridge, page 255.

Sea vegetables

> Add soy sauce. Mix with cooked noodles or salad.
>
> Make into a pie, pages 254.

Beans

> Serve with crackers, tortillas, or chips.
>
> Heat with leftover grains or noodles.
>
> Thin beans, add scallions and more seasoning, and serve over grains, noodles, biscuits, or muffins.
>
> Thin beans to soup consistency and cook noodles or dumplings in it.
>
> Thin beans to soup consistency, add spices, and use to cook polenta.
>
> Make into a spread or dip by puréeing in a blender and adding more seasoning.
>
> Make into casserole, pie, or porridge, pages 253-255.

Fish

> Heat in soup.
>
> Make into a pie, pages 255; or casserole, page 253; or burgers, page 251.

Salads

> Add more of the seasoning that was in the original salad and mix with cooked noodles, grains, or sea vegetables.

Sauces

Serve over vegetables, grains, or noodles.

Serve as a spread or dip.

Make into pie, page 255; or casserole, page 253.

Pickles

Make less salty: Mince finely and mix with a small amount of lemon or ginger juice.

Mince finely and mix into salad or use as a topping for salad in the proportion of 1 part pickle to 4 parts salad. Let stand 15 to 20 minutes before serving.

Make into a condiment: Mince finely and mix with an equal part of minced raw cucumber or celery. Let stand 15 to 20 minutes before serving.

Breads

Serve in soup or with a sauce.

Steam dry or stale bread until soft, 10 to 15 minutes.

Make croutons: Cube bread. Fry in oil, or toast without oil until crisp.

Fruit desserts

Use as a topping for pancakes or muffins.

Use as a filling in muffins, page 207.

Use as an ingredient in cookies, page 231.

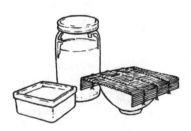

Menu Planning

Overview – Macrobiotic menu planning starts with an emphasis on whole grains, fresh vegetables, and whole beans. These three food categories provide the basis for abundant complex carbohydrates, complete protein, and adequate fiber needed for optimal health.

Macrobiotic teachers from George Ohsawa, Michio Kushi, and Herman Aihara to the numerous other macrobiotic teachers all emphasize the need to eat whole grains. Brown rice, whole wheat, whole corn and corn products, millet, buckwheat, whole oats and rolled oats, barley, and other grains are the primary foods of a macrobiotic diet.

Vegetables and beans are secondary food choices to whole grains. Vegetables are encouraged at each meal, even breakfast, and often in similar proportions as whole grains. Due to the more perishable nature of vegetables, seasonal and local fresh vegetables are encouraged over canned, frozen, or imported varieties. Organically-grown foods are always preferred. Beans complement whole grains to provide complete protein. They often are included daily, but are not stressed as having to be, and are used in lesser proportions to grains.

In addition, other items are included to provide smaller amounts of needed nutrients such as an additional source of fat, whether oil, nuts, seeds, or fish, and a source for minerals such as sea vegetables and high quality sea salt. Fruits are another source of vitamins and enjoyment.

Studying menu planning is a way to learn how to choose good quality foods, both from a theoretical understanding of sound nutrition and from a practical way of how to actually put meals together. This chapter is an introduction to both theoretical and practical menu planning. Use these ideas as a guide in determining your own system of menu planning.

General planning – Practical menu planning is a way to organize your-self and to establish order and consistency. There are four areas of planning outlined in this section: individual meals, and daily, weekly, and seasonal planning. In actual practice they are used together.

I like to start with a weekly plan that takes into account seasonal needs. This might be written or merely thought through. Here is an example of a general weekly winter plan (only a few items are included): buckwheat sometime this week; lentil soup later in the week, perhaps Thursday; noodles on Friday; fish either Friday or Saturday.

Specific planning – After determining a general weekly plan, note which dishes such as beans or bread require soaking or lengthy preparation. You can space the cooking so that major preparations fall on different days or plan to cook all these items on the same day. Each day think over the general plan and confirm or change it depending on time, number of leftovers, and choice of fresh ingredients. Figure out each meal, taking into account daily needs. Note when to soak things and when to start cooking.

To give an example, my general plan called for buckwheat sometime in the week. On Tuesday night, noting there is only enough left-over rice for breakfast, I plan buckwheat for lunch and a new pot of rice for dinner. I will wash the rice and put it on to soak Wednesday morning. On Wednesday night, knowing the general plan is for lentil soup on Thursday, I plan to cook lentils on Thursday in the early morning to allow enough time to cook and serve it for lunch.

Saving time – Planning ahead saves time in the long run; you know what to prepare ahead of time and what to purchase. You also can save time by letting time work for you. Soak rice overnight and cook it early in the morning before going to work. Knead bread in the evening and let it rise overnight; bake it in the morning.

Another way to save time is to cook in quantity, especially dishes such as bread, beans, cooked grains, and pickles that take a long time to prepare. Some vegetables, like winter squash, are usable as leftovers but most vegetables are best when freshly cooked.

Cooking in quantity allows meals to be coordinated. For example, cook polenta one day and have fried polenta slices the next day. Cook extra winter squash to use in filled muffins.

Individual Meal Planning

Full Meals – When preparing a multi-course meal, it is relatively easy to cover all nutritive needs because there are many dishes. Here are some guidelines to help you.

1. Grains and beans – Choose grains and beans that complement each other to create the cornerstone of meals. Use traditional choices such as pinto beans and cornmeal, soup and bread, lentils and brown rice as models.

2. Fish – If serving fish, choose a complementary grain. For example: fried perch with soba; baked salmon with couscous and vegetables; steamed cod with rice salad.

3. Vegetables – Choose vegetables for seasonal support, color, freshness, and complement. Examples: fresh lettuce salad with pinto beans and cornmeal; boiled kale with baked salmon and couscous and vegetables; fresh scallions to garnish soba and fried perch.

4. Soups – Vary the choice of soup. A thick and rich soup such as black bean soup or Russian soup can be a central component, while a light soup such as kombu soup broth for soba can be a complement.

5. Sea Vegetables – If possible, try to include some sort of sea vegetable into each meal, whether a full dish such as hijiki or as an ingredient such as kombu cooked into a bean dish.

6. Oil – Use oil in at least one dish, or include seeds, nuts, or their butters. Adjust the amount of oil per season and for your own needs.

7. Sea salt – Cook sea salt into dishes rather than sprinkling it on food after it has been cooked. Salt changes as it cooks and cooked salt is easier for the body to assimilate. Use soy sauce, umeboshi, or miso to reduce the amount of, or in place of, sea salt if desired.

8. Pickles and tea – Pickles and tea may be served at each meal

if desired. Pickles aid digestion, and tea is soothing after eating.

9. Foods and preparations – Use a variety of preparations and
foods to create balanced menus. For example, avoid baking
everything or serving 100 percent grain on a daily basis.

10. Fancy and simple – Serve only one fancy dish such as a dish
with many ingredients or colors at any meal. Simplify the
rest of the meal.

11. Shapes – A variety of cutting styles makes the meal more
attractive, both overall and within each dish.

12. Textures – A variety of textures make the meal more appealing: creamy soups and sauces, chewy bread, firm vegetables,
crunchy seeds, and crisp salads.

13. Colors – A spectrum of color is available—for example:
green, orange, or yellow vegetables; black sea vegetables;
red, green, or white beans; brown or tan grain. Colors can be
used creatively over the whole meal as well as in each dish.

Simple Meals – When preparing a simple meal it is important to plan
well so that one is satisfied nutritionally with the dishes that are made.
When one cooks a lot of dishes, one can easily cover all the variety one
needs by cooking beans, soup, or sea vegetables along with grains and
vegetables. But when one cooks only one or two dishes it becomes important to pay attention so nothing is left out.

One idea that has worked well for me for years is the idea of "three
categories." The idea is to include all the nutritive groups without having to prepare as many dishes as when preparing a more complex meal.
The first category is "grains," the second category is "vegetables," and
the third category is "everything else." When I am cooking a quick or
simple meal, I'll prepare a grain, a vegetable, and something else that
is not a grain or vegetable. This can be as simple as toasting seeds for
cooked vegetables or making a sauce for pasta. It can be a bowl of pea
soup with whole grain crackers and carrot sticks, or leftover brown rice
scrambled with tofu and other vegetables.

Basic rule of thumb – The building blocks of macrobiotic nutritional theory include complex carbohydrates from grains and beans; protein from beans, fish, and nuts to some degree; and fat from oil, seeds, nuts, fish, and beans to some degree. Fiber, vitamins, and freshness come from vegetables as well as all whole foods. Include complex carbohydrates, proteins, and fats at each meal and consume carbohydrates as the largest group, then proteins, then fats. The amount of vegetables can be equal to the amount of carbohydrates, if desired.

It is important to consume all three major nutritive sources at each meal and to avoid omitting any. I first heard these ideas from Annemarie Colbin and have verified them for myself and family. Satisfaction and long-term health benefits come from a regular daily diet. If any of these three categories is consistently omitted, it is possible to develop deficiencies or to set yourself up for severe cravings. Take care of yourself and include all three major nutrient categories for consistency and stability.

Daily Planning

Number and type of meals – Eating on a consistent schedule can create order and regularity. I like to eat three times a day with a light breakfast, simple lunch, and a fancier dinner. My growing kids like three meals with two snacks in between. While you may choose a different daily plan, try to have one meal more elaborate than the others.

When beginning macrobiotics, all my meals were simple. My diet quickly became boring. When I studied cooking in macrobiotic classes, all my meals became gourmet-style and fancy. My diet became too rich, and cooking too time-consuming. Now, I aim for the middle. One meal each day is bigger and more elaborate than the others.

Daily needs – Everyone has daily needs of various nutrients. Foods commonly used within a macrobiotic diet supply these daily needs, but macrobiotic principles also remind us that individual needs change as conditions change. One day you may feel you need more protein, from fish for example; other days less. Some days more salads or desserts; others more grains.

In planning menus, I like to draw up a minimum daily guideline per person. The following list is based on my current general needs; foods should be added or deleted depending on each person's needs and preferences. For example, when I was pregnant, I tried to have two daily servings of sea vegetables.

> Miso soup – 1 serving
> Another soup (not miso soup) – 1 serving
> Grain – at least 2 servings
> Noodles, bread, or a different grain – 1 serving
> Beans or protein source – 1 to 2 servings
> Sea vegetable – 1 serving
> Dish with oil – 1 serving per meal
> Green vegetable – 1 serving
> Yellow vegetable – 1 serving
> Root vegetable – 1 serving
> Leafy vegetable – 1 serving
> Pickles – 2 servings
> Tea – 2 servings
> Water – throughout the day as needed

Weekly Planning

Cooking schedule – When working, it is necessary to set up a compatible cooking schedule. While working 8:00 to 5:00, Monday through Friday, I often cooked a lot on Saturday and Sunday, had leftovers on Monday and Tuesday, and made simple, quick meals on Wednesday, Thursday, and Friday. When I was home with young children, I cooked each day and tried to vary the menus so the bulk of the cooking was every second or third day. To simplify planning, I had special meals on certain nights: Thursday was noodle night, for instance.

After 25 years of cooking macrobiotic meals, I have used one thing consistently in menu planning: the plain spiral notebook. Every Sunday our family has a weekly meeting during which we review schedules, appointments, and recreational activities, and plan for menus we want to eat. I record it all in the notebook and base the menus accordingly, cooking more variety and quantity on the days when I can be in the kitchen and preparing quick menus and utilizing leftovers on days when it is more rushed.

Food variety – Grains and vegetables are served daily, yet they can be varied in the weekly schedule. Rice can be varied each time by mixing it with a different grain or with beans. Between pots of rice, prepare other grains, noodles, or quick breads. Vary green vegetables during the week by using different kinds such as cabbage, kale, and broccoli. Vary the dishes by using different preparations such as layering, simmering, and stir-frying.

Weekly food guidelines – For foods that are not served daily, here are general weekly suggestions per person. As in the daily food guideline, this list can change depending on personal needs and preferences. For example, the need and choice for animal protein varies considerably among individuals. Annemarie Colbin, Ph.D., suggests increasing protein consumption if one has cravings for sweets—this can signal a protein deficiency.

> Nuts, seeds, or sauce – 2 to 3 servings.
> Fish or egg – 1 serving each week in the winter (men and growing children 2 servings); 1 serving every other week in the summer.
> Raw salad – 2 servings in the summer.
> Dessert – 1 to 2 servings (growing children daily).

Seasonal Planning

Yin and yang of seasons   Summer is considered more yang (hotter) than winter, and summer menus should be more yin (cooler) than winter menus. Likewise, winter menus should be more yang than summer menus. Spring and fall are in the middle, so the menus are moderately yin and yang. Yet, spring menus can be slightly more yin because summer approaches, and fall menus can be slightly more yang because winter approaches. As seasons change, menus change both in the specific foods and the ways they are prepared.

Seasonal and local foods – Foods comprise the qualities of the season and the location in which they grow. If you garden or have a local farmer's market it is easy to identify what vegetables are locally grown. If not, think of summer vegetables as quicker-grown vegetables such as cucumbers, summer squash, and lettuces. Winter vegetables are those that keep well, including roots and winter squashes. Seasonal vegetables vary from area to area depending on many factors, from elevation to rainfall to soil type. Explore what grows in your area!

Seasonal variations in procedures – Any procedure can be used at any time of the year; you can boil, sauté, pressure cook, bake, and pickle all year around. Yet for some dishes, certain procedures are more appropriate during a given season than others.

Food	Summer	Winter
vegetables	raw	baked
miso soup	boiled	sautéed/boiled
pickles	brine	pressed

Of course, procedures may be chosen for reasons of balance or other considerations. You may wish to serve raw salad or fruit to balance turkey at Thanksgiving, for example.

Other seasonal modifications – Amounts of sea salt, water, oil, and length of cooking time can be adjusted as the seasons change. For example, increase the proportion of water to rice in the summer and use a smaller proportion in the winter. Use less miso in miso soup in the summer and more in the winter.

Flexibility and adaptability – While all these ideas have been useful to me and my family over the years, none is a hard fast rule. All of these ideas are guidelines to help form wholesome meals. Study, cook, and above all have fun.

Menus

This section includes food lists and several categories of sample menus. Beginning Menus includes familiar foods prepared in simple ways. Menus for Seven Consecutive Days shows a week's worth of meals and how to use leftovers.

Each item is followed by the page number of the recipe. Variations of recipes or procedures have been included in parentheses. An approximate time for preparation of each meal is noted under the last item. Soaking time and any required leftovers are also listed. All menus may include store-bought or homemade pickles. Bancha twig tea, page 244, may be served at any meal.

Menu Suggestions

Breakfast – Try a simple light breakfast of soup, if desired, and grain. Ideas for breakfast include:

> Miso soup.
> Soft-cooked grain such as oatmeal, rice, creamed cereals, or porridge of leftover grain.
> Topping for grain such as roasted seeds or sea vegetables or sesame seed condiments.
> Breads, muffins, toast, pancakes, waffles.
> Spreads or sauces for breads.
> Granola and grain milk.
> Egg dishes.
> Tea.

Lunch or supper – Ideas for a simple meal of grain, vegetable, and one other dish include.

> Any grain dish.
> Any vegetable dish or grain and vegetable combination.
> Simple vegetable, bean, or miso soup if not served at breakfast.
> Sea vegetable dishes.
> Simple bean dishes, or tofu or tempeh dishes.
> Condiments of roasted sea vegetables or seeds.
> Bread, toast, muffins, spreads.
> Bran pickles.
> Simple salads or noodle dishes.
> Tea.

Dinner – For the largest meal of the day, add soup, beans, or whatever else is desired to the basic menu of grain and vegetables. Ideas for dinner include:

> Any grain dish.
> Any vegetable dish or grain and vegetable combination.
> Noodle dishes.
> Fancy soups with dumplings, creamy ingredients, flour, fish.
> Bean dishes.
> Fish or egg dishes.
> Rich sauces with nuts.
> Pressed salads and pickles.
> Pan-fried dishes.
> Desserts.
> Tea.

Good grain and bean combinations – Any of these ideas can serve as a base on which to build a meal.

> Rice with roasted seeds, azuki beans, pinto beans, black beans, lentils, or split peas.
> Millet with chickpeas, lentils, tempeh, or dulse.
> Buckwheat with tahini sauce, scallions, lentils, or tofu.
> Oatmeal with roasted sunflower seeds or dulse.
> Polenta, or cornbread with pinto beans, black beans, or lentils.
> Bulgur with chickpeas or tahini sauce.
> Creamed cereals with miso vegetables.
> Udon or buckwheat noodles with clear kombu broths and garnishes. (More ideas in noodle chapter.)
> Whole wheat noodles with nut butter sauces.

Quick and Easy Foods

Easiest foods to prepare – The following foods are the easiest ones from each food group. Note that some may be more involved than foods listed in other food groups. For example, it is easier to make salt brine pickles than bran pickles but it is easier to make a salad than salt brine pickles.

Grains – Boiled grain; soaked, unsoaked using cold water, unsoaked using hot water.

Noodles – Noodles served with a sauce or cooked into soup.

Vegetables – Any vegetables simmered, layered, or baked. Freshly picked and young vegetables are easier to cut and prepare than older vegetables.

Salads – Raw salads and mixed dressings.

Soups – Stews, boiled vegetable soups, soups with noodles.

Beans – Boiled bean dishes.

Sea vegetables – Kombu used in bean dishes, agar used in kanten gelled desserts.

Sauces and condiments – Nut butter sauces, spreads, nuts or seeds roasted on top of the stove or oven.

Pickles and pressed salads – Salt brine pickles, salt brine pressed salads.

Fish and egg – Baked or broiled fish, scrambled eggs, eggs in baked goods.

Breads – Batter breads, muffins, biscuits, pancakes, dumplings.

Desserts and snacks – Fruit sauces, stewed dried fruit, grain puddings, drop cookies, trail mixes.

Beverages – Bancha twig tea, juices.

Leftovers – Grains sautéed with tofu and vegetables, porridge, grain puddings.

Foods that can be prepared in small quantities – The following foods are the easiest from each food group to make in a small amount. These are especially useful when cooking for one.

Grains – Millet, oatmeal, polenta, bulgur, rice cream, hard-kernelled grains (rice, oats, wheat) in a small pressure cooker.

Noodles – All noodles.

Vegetables – All vegetables and procedures except baked.

Salads – All salads.

Soups – Boiled vegetable soups, sautéed vegetable soups, kombu soups, instant soups.

Beans – Tofu, tempeh, lentils, azuki beans, split peas.

Sea vegetables – Roasted dulse, wakame, or nori.

Sauces and condiments – Mixed sauces, clear sauces, nut butter sauces, nuts and seeds roasted on top of the stove.

Pickles and pressed salads – Pressed salads with salt brine or soy sauce brine.

Fish and egg – Pan-fried, broiled, or steamed fish; scrambled eggs.

Breads – Pancakes, biscuits, muffins.

Desserts and snacks – Sautéed fruit, fruit in clear sauce, fruit with sauce, couscous puddings, popcorn, trail mixes.

Beverages – Bancha twig tea, juices.

Leftovers – Grains sautéed with tofu and vegetables, burgers, porridge, fried grain slices, most suggestions listed on pages 256-258.

Quickest foods to prepare – These foods can be prepared in 30 minutes or less. Use these ideas when in a hurry or when unexpected guests arrive.

Grains – Boiled millet, oatmeal, bulgur, polenta, couscous.

Noodles – All noodles.

Vegetables – Pressure cooked, stir-fried, sautéed with or without water, layered, or simmered vegetables. Some vegetables such as greens require more time to wash and some cutting styles, for example, dicing, take more time to cut.

Salads – All salads and dressings.

Soups – Boiled soups, pressure-cooked soups, instant soups, kombu soups.

Beans – Tofu, tempeh dishes.

Sea vegetables – Dulse or wakame salads, roasted nori, dulse, or wakame.

Sauces and condiments – Mixed sauces, clear sauces, nut butter sauces, miso sauces, tofu sauces, nuts and seeds roasted on top of the stove or in the oven.

Fish and egg – All except baked fish with vegetables.

Breads – Dumplings, pancakes, waffles.

Desserts and snacks – Sautéed fruit, fruit in clear sauce, fruit with sauce, couscous puddings, popcorn, trail mixes.

Beverages – Bancha twig tea, juices.

Leftovers – Burgers, porridge, fried grain slices, most suggestions listed on pages 256-258.

Beginning Menus

Boiled oatmeal, page 60. (This is a breakfast menu.)
Stewed prunes, page 220.
Roasted sunflower seeds, pages 183-184.
Time: 30 minutes.

Split pea soup, page 146.
Boiled sautéed bulgur, page 64.
Simmered carrots, page 98.
Oat crisp, page 209.
Time: 1½ hours.

Cabbage noodle soup, page 115.
Boiled millet, page 59.
Winter squash and carrots, page 83.
Roasted almonds with soy sauce, comments pages 183-184.
Applesauce, page 221.
Time: 60 minutes.

New England-style vegetable stew, page 107.
Boiled brown rice, page 58.
Cornmeal biscuits, page 208.
Nut butter sauce (use tahini), page 178.
Time: 1½ hours.

Kitchen soup, page 108.
Whole wheat noodles, page 75.
– Serve cooked noodles in soup.
Baked winter squash, page 81.
Sautéed tempeh with mushrooms, page 153.
Time 1½ hours.

Scrambled tofu with millet, page 148.
– Requires leftover millet.
Tossed lettuce salad of choice, page 163.
Olive oil and umeboshi vinegar dressing, page 167.
Time: 15 minutes.

Quick Menus

Whole wheat noodles, page 75.
Simmered broccoli and carrots, variation, page 97.
Tofu and tahini sauce, page 182; or Nut butter sauce, use tahini,
    page 178.
– Serve desired sauce on top of noodles and vegetables.
Time: 30 minutes.

Boiled quinoa, page 63.
Butternut squash and kale, page 88.
– Serve vegetables over grain.
Roasted sunflower or pumpkin seeds, pages 183-184.
Sautéed apples, page 219.
Time: 30 minutes.

Pan-fried tempeh, page 152.
Whole wheat bread, page 204 or 205, or store-bought bread.
Pressed cabbage pickles, page 195, or store-bought sauerkraut.
– Make a sandwich of tempeh, bread, pickles, and lettuce and
    sprouts as desired.
Couscous and squash pudding, page 227.
Time: 30 minutes. Requires leftover winter squash for pudding.
    Bread and pickles already made or store-bought.

Instant orange soup, page 106.
Grain burgers (use brown rice), page 251.
Lettuce, cucumber, and sunflower salad, page 164.
Soy sauce dressing (use lemon juice), page 166.
– Serve dressing separately for use on salad.
Time: 30 minutes. Requires leftover rice for burgers.

Soba or udon noodles, page 75.
Clear sauce or mushroom sauce, pages 174-175.
Nori matchsticks, page 134.
– Serve sauce over noodles and garnish with nori.
Turnips, rutabagas, and carrots, page 86.
Time: 30 minutes.

Summer Menus

Corn and green bean chowder, page 118.
Rice salad, page 171.
Peach and apple kanten, page 228.
Time: 45 minutes. Requires leftover rice for salad and letting
    kanten set 1½ hours.

Arame with green beans and carrots, page 128.
Whole wheat ribbon noodles, page 75.
– Mix noodles with arame, see comments under hijiki, page 127.
Corn on the cob, page 97.
Tossed lettuce, celery, and radish salad, variation, page 163.
Umeboshi and scallion dressing, page 169.
– Mix dressing and toss with salad.
Time: 45 minutes.

Creamy cauliflower soup with dumplings, page 110.
Brown rice combination with barley, page 68.
Summer squash, page 92.
Lettuce, cucumber, and scallion pressed salad, page 193.
Time: 60 to 75 minutes. Requires soaking rice and barley for 4 or
    more hours and pressing salad for 1 hour.

Black turtle bean soup, page 143.
Boiled brown rice, page 58, optional.
Cornmeal batter bread, page 206.
Cucumber and avocado salad, page 165.
Time: 2 hours. Requires soaking beans for 6 to 8 hours and letting
    the bread rise in the sun for 3 to 4 hours.

Steamed cod, page 159.
Millet with vegetables, page 66.
Green beans with almonds, page 100.
Simple lemon cake with glaze, page 238.
Berry sauce (use strawberries), page 223.
– Serve strawberries on cake.
Time: 45 minutes.

Winter Menus

Hearty winter miso soup with millet, comments pages 120-121.
Buckwheat muffins, page 207.
Nut butter spread or quick hummus, page 187.
– Use tahini and scallions.
Time: 1½ hours.

Brown rice combination with azuki beans, page 69.
Baked butternut squash, page 80 or 81.
Broccoli, page 97.
Roasted pumpkin or sunflower seeds, pages 183-184.
Time: 60 to 75 minutes. Requires soaking rice for 6 to 8 hours.

Golden soup, page 113.
Boiled roasted buckwheat, page 62.
Nut butter sauce, low-fat, page 178, use tahini.
– Serve sauce on buckwheat; garnish with scallions.
Cabbage, page 92.
Oatmeal and walnut cookies, page 230.
Time: 60 minutes.

Lentil soup, page 140.
Fried polenta slices, page 252.
Pressure-cooked rice, optional, page 68.
Kale, page 103.
Onion or scallion miso, page 91.
– Serve on polenta.
Time: 2 hours. Requires cooked polenta and soaking rice, if used,
    for 6 to 8 hours.

Kombu clear soup with lemon, comments, page 124.
Baked brown rice, page 71.
Pan-fried perch, page 155, or baked trout, page 157.
Dulse with rutabagas, page 129.
Brussels sprouts, cauliflower, and carrots, page 84.
Apricot pudding, page 224.
Time: 75 to 90 minutes.

Menus for Seven Consecutive Days

These menus are included as an example of a week's menus. They show how to use leftovers, how to use cooking time efficiently and economically, and how to provide variety. For reheating leftovers, see page 250. Note that quantities of some dishes are prepared for more than one meal. The number of meals' worth of each dish is indicated following the final page number.

All menus may include store-bought or homemade pickles. Bancha twig tea, page 240, may be served at any meal, also.

Sunday breakfast

> Boiled oatmeal, page 60.
> Roasted sunflower seeds, page 183 or 184.
> Stewed apricots or prunes, page 220.
> Time 30 minutes.

Sunday lunch

> Boiled brown rice, roasted, page 62, for 3 meals.
> Hijiki with tempeh, page 127, for 2 meals.
> Stir-fried yellow squash, cabbage, and carrots, page 88.
> Time: 60 to 70 minutes.

Sunday dinner

> Leftover rice from Sunday lunch.
> Creamy leek soup, page 117, for 3 meals.
> Mustard greens, page 92.
> Apple crisp, page 218, for 2 meals.
> Time: 60 to 75 minutes.

Monday breakfast

> Instant orange soup, page 106, use miso.
> Quinoa, page 63, for 2 meals.
> Time: 30 minutes.

Monday lunch

Leftover Quinoa from Monday breakfast, fried with onion and garlic, page 88 and 256.
Leftover Hijiki with tempeh from Sunday lunch.
Kale, page 103.
Time: 15 minutes.

Monday dinner

Leftover Creamy leek soup from Sunday dinner.
Pasta, page 75, for 2 meals; served with Tofu and tahini sauce, page 182.
Layered summer squash and green beans, page 83.
Leftover Apple crisp from Sunday dinner.
Time: 30 minutes. Prepare Pressed cabbage pickles, page 195, and soak pinto beans, pages 135 and 143, for 3 meals.

Tuesday breakfast

Grain and vegetable porridge using leftover rice from Sunday lunch, leftover creamy leek soup from Sunday dinner, and fresh miso, page 255.
Time: 10 minutes. Soak rice, pages 56 and 58, for 3 meals.

Tuesday lunch

Leftover Pasta from Monday dinner, fried with tofu, onions, garlic, and carrots, variation, page 148.
Collard greens with cornmeal, page 85.
Roasted pumpkin seeds, pages 183-184.
Time: 30 minutes.

Tuesday dinner

Spring or summer winter miso soup, page 121, for 3 meals.
Boiled long grain brown rice, page 58.
Mexican (pinto) beans, page 143.
Green lettuce salad, page 163, with Avocado dressing, page 167.
Time: 1½ hours.

Wednesday breakfast

Leftover Miso soup from Tuesday dinner.
Leftover Brown rice from Tuesday dinner. Serve rice in soup.
Time: 10 minutes. Soak Rice and whole rye combination, pages 56 and 68, for 2 meals.

Wednesday lunch

Leftover beans and rice, heat together with scallions.
– Serve with store-bought corn tortillas or corn chips and sauce.
Nut butter sauce (use tahini) page 178.
Green lettuce salad, page 163.
Olive oil and umeboshi vinegar dressing, page 167.
Time: 15 minutes.

Wednesday dinner

Pressure-cooked rice and rye, page 68.
Leftover Mexican (pinto) beans from Tuesday dinner.
Cabbage, carrot, and celery "cooked salad," page 102.
– Serve with dressing of choice
Clear soup with scallions and soy sauce, using water from cooked
   vegetables, see comments, page 101.

Thursday breakfast

Leftover Miso soup from Tuesday dinner.
Rice pudding, page 224, use rice and rye from Wednesday dinner.
Time: 15 minutes. Soak chickpeas, pages 135 and 147, for 2
   meals.

Thursday lunch

Soba noodles, page 75, with scallion and nori garnishes.
Specialty dressing, page 167.
Roasted almonds, chopped, page 183 or 184.
Broccoli, page 97.
Time: 20 minutes.

Thursday dinner

Pressure-cooked millet, page 69, for 2 meals.
Chickpea sauce, page 147.
– Serve Chickpea sauce over millet.
Pressed cabbage pickles, made on Monday.
Time: 2 hours. Set half of millet into loaf pan.

Friday breakfast

Cleansing miso soup, page 119, for 2 meals.
Steel-cut oats or oatmeal, page 60.
Time: 40 minutes.

Friday lunch

Fried millet slices, page 252
Stir-fried broccoli, carrots, and tofu, page 89, variation with ginger
    and sauce, see comments.
Nori with soy sauce, page 130.
Roasted sunflower seeds, page 183 or 184.
Time: 30 minutes.

Friday dinner

Kombu clear soup with Chinese cabbage, tofu, and scallions, varia-
    tion, page 123.
Pan-fried perch, page 155.
Udon noodles, page 75.
– Serve soup over noodles and fish in one bowl.
Winter squash, page 99, for 2 meals.
Time: 60 minutes. Soak rice, pages 56 and 58, for 2 meals. Knead
    Whole wheat bread, page 204, and let rise overnight.

Saturday breakfast

Leftover miso soup from Friday breakfast.
Buckwheat pancakes, page 210.
Raisin sauce, page 220, to top pancakes.
Time: 30 minutes. Bake bread for 1 to 1½ hours, page 204.

Saturday lunch

Boiled short grain brown rice, page 58.
Lentil soup, page 140.
Fresh bread.
Walnut miso, page 179.
Green lettuce salad, page 163, or kale, page 103.
Time: 60 minutes.

Saturday dinner

Chickpea soup using leftover Chickpea sauce from Thursday din-
    ner, see ideas for beans page 257.
Leftover Brown rice from Saturday lunch.
– Serve soup over rice.
Broccoli, page 97.
Whole wheat muffins with squash filling, using leftover squash
    from Friday dinner, see comments, page 207.
Time: 45 minutes.

Suggested Readings

Macrobiotic Books

Aihara, Herman – *Acid and Alkaline*, George Ohsawa Macrobiotic Foundation, Oroville, 1986.

Aihara, Herman – *Basic Macrobiotics, Revised*, George Ohsawa Macrobiotic Foundation, Oroville, 1998.

Albert, Rachel – *Cooking with Rachel*, George Ohsawa Macrobiotic Foundation, Oroville, 1989.

Baum, Lenore – *Lenore's Natural Cuisine*, Culinary Publications, Asheville, 2000.

Baum, Lenore – *Sublime Soups*, Culinary Publications, Asheville, 2002.

Belleme, John and Jan – *The Miso Book*, Square One Publishers, Garden City Park, 2004.

Colbin, Annemarie – *Food and Healing*, Ballantine Books, New York, 1986.

Colbin, Annemarie – *Food and Our Bones*, Ballantine Books, New York, 1998.

Ferré, Carl – *Pocket Guide to Macrobiotics*, Crossing Press, Berkeley, 1997.

Gagné, Steve – *Energetics of Food*, Spiral Sciences, Santa Fe, 1990.

Heidenry, Carolyn – *Making the Transition to a Macrobiotic Diet*, Avery, New York, 1984.

Henkel, Pamela and Lee Koch – *As Easy As 1, 2, 3*, George Ohsawa Macrobiotic Foundation, Oroville, 1990.

Kushi, Aveline, with Alex Jack – *Complete Guide to Macrobiotic Cooking*, Warner Books, New York, 1985.

Kushi, Michio, with Alex Jack – *Cancer Prevention Diet, revised*, St. Martin's Griffin, New York, 1993.

Kushi, Michio, and Jack, Alex – *Macrobiotic Path to Total Health*, Ballantine Books, New York, 2003.

Kushi, Michio – *Macrobiotic Way, 3rd Edition*, Avery, New York, 1985.

Kushi, Michio – *Your Face Never Lies*, Avery, New York, 1983.

Lawson, Margaret, with Monte, Tom – *Naturally Healthy Gourmet*, George Ohsawa Macrobiotic Foundation, Oroville, 1994.

McCarty, Meredith – *American Macrobiotic Cuisine*, Avery, New York, 1986.

McCarty, Meredith – *Sweet and Natural*, St. Martin's Griffin, New York, 1999.

Ohashi, Wataru, with Monte, Tom – *Reading the Body*, Penguin Compass, New York, 1991.

Ohsawa, George, edited by Carl Ferré – *Essential Ohsawa*, George Ohsawa Macrobiotic Foundation, Oroville, 1994.

Ohsawa, George – *Macrobiotic Guidebook for Living*, George Ohsawa Macrobiotic Foundation, Oroville, 1985.

Ohsawa, George, English version by William Dufty – *You Are All Sanpaku*, Citadel Press, New York, 2002.

Ohsawa, George – *Zen Macrobiotics, Unabridged Edition*, George Ohsawa Macrobiotic Foundation, Oroville, 1995.

Pirello, Christina – *Cook Your Way to the Life You Want*, HP Books, New York, 1999.

Pirello, Christina – *Cooking the Whole Foods Way*, HP Books, New York, 1997.

Pirello, Christina – *Everything You Always Wanted to Know about Whole Foods*, HP Books, New York, 2004.

Pirello, Christina – *Glow: A Prescription for Radiant Health and Beauty*, HP Books, New York, 2001.

Porter, Jessica – *Hip Chick's Guide to Macrobiotics*, Avery, New York, 2005.

Rivière, Françoise – *#7 Diet*, George Ohsawa Macrobiotic Foundation, Chico, 2005.

Rowland, Natalie Buckley – *Valley of Maize*, George Ohsawa Macrobiotic Foundation, Oroville, 1998.

Stanchich, Lino – *Macrobiotic Healing Secrets*, Healthy Products, Asheville, 2000.

Stanchich, Lino – *Power Eating Program*, Healthy Products, Asheville, 1989.

Turner, Kristina – *Self-Healing Cookbook*, Earthtones Press, Vashon Island, 1987.

Varona, Verne – *Nature's Cancer-Fighting Foods*, Reward Books, New York, 2001.

Waxman, Denny – *The Great Life Handbook*, Denny Waxman Enterprises, Philadelphia, 2002.

Weber, Marcea – *Naturally Sweet Desserts*, Avery, New York, 1990.

Willmont, Dennis – *Fat Chance: Surviving the Cholesterol Controversy and Beyond*, Willmountain Press, Marshfield, MA, 2006.

Wood, Rebecca – *New Whole Foods Encyclopedia*, Penguin Compass, New York, 1999.

Wood, Rebecca – *The Splendid Grain*, William Morrow and Company, New York, 1999

Using Other Cookbooks

In general – You don't need to throw out all your favorite cookbooks if you wish to cook macrobiotically. Use and adapt them to fit your needs. Here are tips for using vegetarian, ethnic, or traditional cookbooks.

Compatible recipes – Look for a recipe that can be used without having to change the most important ingredients. For example, changing a recipe of pot roast and potatoes to one of brown rice and carrots is not reasonable. Changing a recipe of pizza with canned foods to pizza with fresh cooked foods is feasible.

Interpreting recipes: easy or difficult – Read the recipe to see what steps are involved and how much skill and which utensils are needed. A recipe with many steps and utensils is harder and more time consuming than one with fewer steps and utensils. Skills such as rolling out dough, crimping edges together, and frosting a cake can be difficult to perform the first time.

Adapting recipes – Change the recipe by substituting good quality alternatives for undesired foods. Use oil instead of margarine, whole grain pasta for white pasta, arrowroot powder for cornstarch. When a recipe requires sugar, milk, or meat, it is harder to adapt, but not impossible. Substitute maple syrup or rice syrup for sugar and reduce the quantity of liquid in the recipe; use soymilk or rice milk in place of milk. Meat substitutions require creative cooking techniques and replacements such as seitan, which is not covered in this book.

Change recipes by combining or adding procedures. If the recipe calls for tofu, make sure the tofu will be cooked at some point in preparation. For example, if making a blended tofu dip, boil the tofu before blending to freshen and make more digestible.

When changing recipes, maintain the consistency to create a similar product. Check the ratios of the original recipe for liquids, fats and oils, and salt. Make the altered recipe similar in texture and presentation.

Balance – Check recipe for balance considerations for extreme yin items or yang items. For example, if a recipe calls for ginger juice and sake over mushrooms and omits salt, change it and add soy sauce for better balance. If a cooked fruit recipe has no salt, cook with a pinch of salt. If a fish recipe has salt or soy sauce without any yin quality, add a yin factor such as ginger juice. This step adds to the success or failure of the recipe and to the satisfaction of the meal.

A Word on Supplies and Suppliers

Many stores carry the foods and supplies needed for macrobiotic cooking. There are several mail order companies and distributors. The publisher of this book maintains a current list of suppliers and a catalog of macrobiotic books. Contact the George Ohsawa Macrobiotic Foundation, PO Box 3998, Chico, CA 95927-3998; 800-232-2372; 530-566-9765; 530-566-9768 (fax); *gomf@earthlink.net* for the most recent information.

Index